A Text Book of

MEDICINAL CHEMISTRY - I

Second Year B. Pharm., Semester IV

As Per PCI Regulations

Dr. Chandrashekhar Narajji
M. Pharm., Ph.D.
Professor and Head,
Pharmaceutical Chemistry Deptt.,
Mallige College of Pharmacy,
Bangalore.

Mrs. Vibha Chandan Patil
M.Pharm.
Associate Professor,
Pharmaceutical Chemsitry Deptt.,
Mallige College of Pharmacy,
Bangalore.

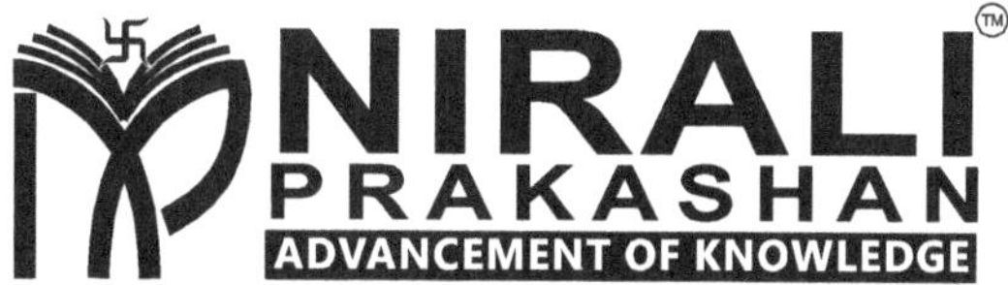

N4358

Medicinal Chemistry - I   **ISBN 978-93-88897-57-0**

Second Edition : February 2020

© : **Authors**

Published By :

NIRALI PRAKASHAN

Abhyudaya Pragati, 1312, Shivaji Nagar,
Off J.M. Road, PUNE – 411005
Tel - (020) 25512336/37/39, Fax - (020) 25511379
Email : niralipune@pragationline.com

➢ ## DISTRIBUTION CENTRES

PUNE

Nirali Prakashan : 119, Budhwar Peth, Jogeshwari Mandir Lane, Pune 411002, Maharashtra
Tel : (020) 2445 2044, 66022708
Email : bookorder@pragationline.com, niralilocal@pragationline.com

Nirali Prakashan : S. No. 28/27, Dhyari, Near Pari Company, Pune 411041
Tel : (020) 24690204 Fax : (020) 24690316
Email : dhyari@pragationline.com, bookorder@pragationline.com

MUMBAI

Nirali Prakashan : 385, S.V.P. Road, Rasdhara Co-op. Hsg. Society Ltd.,
Girgaum, Mumbai 400004, Maharashtra
Tel : (022) 2385 6339 / 2386 9976, Fax : (022) 2386 9976
Email : niralimumbai@pragationline.com

➢ ## DISTRIBUTION BRANCHES

JALGAON

Nirali Prakashan : 34, V. V. Golani Market, Navi Peth, Jalgaon 425001,
Maharashtra, Tel : (0257) 222 0395, Mob : 94234 91860
Email : niralijalgoan@pragationline.com

KOLHAPUR

Nirali Prakashan : New Mahadvar Road, Kedar Plaza, 1st Floor Opp. IDBI Bank
Kolhapur 416 012, Maharashtra. Mob : 9850046155
Email : niralikolhapur@pragationline.com

NAGPUR

Nirali Prakashan : Above Maratha Mandir, Shop No. 3, First Floor,
Rani Jhanshi Square, Sitabuldi, Nagpur 440012, Maharashtra
Tel : (0712) 254 7129; Email : niralinagpur@pragationline.com

DELHI

Nirali Prakashan : 4593/15, Basement, Agarwal Lane, Ansari Road, Daryaganj
Near Times of India Building, New Delhi 110002 Mob : 08505972553
Email : niralidelhi@pragationline.com

BANGALURU

Nirali Prakashan : Maitri Ground Floor, Jaya Apartments, No. 99, 6th Cross, 6th Main,
Malleswaram, Bengaluru 560003, Karnataka; Mob : 9449043034
Email : niralibangalore@pragationline.com

Other Branches : Hyderabad, Chennai

niralipune@pragationline.com | www.pragationline.com
Also find us on www.facebook.com/niralibooks

Acknowledgement

We are indebted to Dr. M. D. Karvekar for reviewing the entire manuscript and for making numerous valuable comments.

Authors extend their immense thanks towards Mallige Education foundation our beloved chairman Dr. A.C. Sreeram and Mr. N. Ramesh (General Manager), Principal and Staff of Mallige College of Pharmacy for their great support.

Preface

As per the need of students and instructors, we have been engaged in writing and compiling the data based on Pharmacy Council of Indian regulated syllabus. It gives us immense pleasure to introduce "Text Book of Medicinal Chemistry - I". This book has been designed and arranged to provide the basic knowledge of chemistry of drugs, drug interaction and drug metabolism. The content is focused on synthesis and structure-activity relationship of drugs which enable determination of chemical group responsible for evoking a target biological effect in the organism.

Book is written in a simple and comprehensive manner along with the structure, schematic diagrams and tables that clearly demonstrate core concept of medicinal chemistry. The authentic text of the book will definitely furnish exhaustive information to the students with impressively and user-friendly style.

The contents of the book are structured as per Pharmacy Council of India regulated syllabus and will be more useful to undergraduate students pursuing career in pharmaceutical science in India.

We will be highly thankful to our publishers Mr. Dineshbhai Furia, Mr. Jignesh Furia of Nirali Prakashan and the staff members especially Mr. Malik Shaikh, Mr. Kiran Velankar, Mrs. Varsha Bodake, Ms. Chaitali Takle and Mrs. Yojana Deshpande for immense support and patience.

We will be grateful to all the students, teachers and readers for their constructive suggestions to improve the quality of contents of this book. The suggestions from all the readers will be highly appreciated and will be incorporated in the next edition.

Dr. Chandrashekhar Narajji

Mrs. Vibha Chandan Patil

Syllabus

Unit - I   **10 Hours**

Introduction to Medicinal Chemistry

History and Development of Medicinal Chemistry

Physicochemical Properties in relation to Biological Action

Ionization, Solubility, Partition Coefficient, Hydrogen bonding, Protein binding, Chelation, Bioisosterism, Optical and Geometrical isomerism.

Drug Metabolism

Drug metabolism principles- Phase I and Phase II.

Factors affecting drug metabolism including stereochemical aspects.

Unit - II   **10 Hours**

Drugs acting on Autonomic Nervous System

Adrenergic Neurotransmitters:

Biosynthesis and catabolism of catecholamine.

Adrenergic receptors (Alpha & Beta) and their distribution.

Sympathomimetic agents: SAR of Sympathomimetic agents

Direct acting: Nor-epinephrine, Epinephrine, Phenylephrine*, Dopamine, Methyldopa, Clonidine, Dobutamine, Isoproterenol, Terbutaline, Salbutamol*, Bitolterol, Naphazoline, Oxymetazoline and Xylometazoline.

Indirect acting agents: Hydroxyamphetamine, Pseudoephedrine, Propylhexedrine.

Agents with mixed mechanism: Ephedrine, Metaraminol.

Adrenergic Antagonists:

Alpha adrenergic blockers: Tolazoline*, Phentolamine, Phenoxybenzamine, Prazosin, Dihydroergotamine, Methysergide.

Beta adrenergic blockers: SAR of beta blockers, Propranolol*, Metibranolol, Atenolol, Betazolol, Bisoprolol, Esmolol, Metoprolol, Labetolol, Carvedilol.

Unit - III   **10 Hours**

Cholinergic Neurotransmitters:

Biosynthesis and catabolism of acetylcholine.

Cholinergic receptors (Muscarinic and Nicotinic) and their distribution.

Parasympathomimetic agents: SAR of Parasympathomimetic agents

Direct acting agents: Acetylcholine, Carbachol*, Bethanechol, Methacholine, Pilocarpine.

Indirect acting/Cholinesterase inhibitors (Reversible and Irreversible): Physostigmine, Neostigmine*, Pyridostigmine, Edrophonium chloride, Tacrine hydrochloride, Ambenonium chloride, Isofluorphate, Echothiophate iodide, Parathion, Malathion.

Cholinesterase reactivator: Pralidoxime chloride.

Cholinergic blocking agents: SAR of cholinolytic agents

Solanaceous alkaloids and analogues: Atropine sulphate, Hyoscyamine sulphate, Scopolamine hydrobromide, Homatropinehydrobromide, Ipratropium bromide*.

Synthetic cholinergic blocking agents: Tropicamide, Cyclopentolate hydrochloride, Clidinium bromide, Dicyclomine hydrochloride*, Glycopyrrolate, Methantheline bromide, Propantheline bromide, Benztropinemesylate, Orphenadrine citrate, Biperidine hydrochloride, Procyclidine hydrochloride*, Tridihexethyl chloride, Isopropamide iodide, Ethopropazine hydrochloride.

Unit - IV   **08 Hours**
Drugs Acting on Central Nervous System
A. Sedatives and Hypnotics:

Benzodiazepines: SAR of Benzodiazepines, Chlordiazepoxide, Diazepam*, Oxazepam, Chlorazepate, Lorazepam, Alprazolam, Zolpidem

Barbiturtes: SAR of barbiturates, Barbital*, Phenobarbital, Mephobarbital, Amobarbital, Butabarbital, Pentobarbital, Secobarbital

Miscelleneous:

Amides and imides: Glutethimide.

Alcohol and their carbamate derivatives: Meprobamate, Ethchlorvynol.

Aldehydes and their derivatives: Triclofos sodium, Paraldehyde.

B. Antipsychotics

Phenothiazines: SAR of Phenothiazines - Promazine hydrochloride, Chlorpromazine hydrochloride*, Triflupromazine, Thioridazine hydrochloride, Piperacetazine hydrochloride, Prochlorperazine maleate, Trifluoperazine hydrochloride.

Ring Analogues of Phenothiazines: Chlorprothixene, Thiothixene, Loxapine succinate, Clozapine.

Flurobuterophenones: Haloperidol, Droperidol, Risperidone.

Beta amino ketones: Molindone hydrochloride.

Benzamides: Sulpieride.

C. Anticonvulsants: SAR of anticonvulsants, mechanism of anticonvulsant action

Barbiturates: Phenobarbitone, Methabarbital.

Hydantoins: Phenytoin*, Mephenytoin, Ethotoin

Oxazolidinediones: Trimethadione, Paramethadione

Succinimides: Phensuximide, Methsuximide, Ethosuximide*

Urea and Monoacylureas: Phenacemide, Carbamazepine*

Benzodiazepines: Clonazepam

Miscellaneous: Primidone, Valproic acid, Gabapentin, Felbamate

Unit – V   **07 Hours**

Drugs Acting on Central Nervous System

General Anesthetics:

   Inhalation Anesthetics: Halothane*, Methoxyflurane, Enflurane, Sevoflurane, Isoflurane, Desflurane.

   Ultra short acting barbitutrates: Methohexital sodium*, Thiamylal sodium, Thiopental sodium.

   Dissociative Anesthetics: Ketamine hydrochloride.*

Narcotic and Non-narcotic Analgesics

   Morphine and Related Drugs: SAR of Morphine analogues, Morphine sulphate, Codeine, Meperidine hydrochloride, Anilerdine hydrochloride, Diphenoxylate hydrochloride, Loperamide hydrochloride, Fentanyl citrate*, Methadone hydrochloride*, Propoxyphene hydrochloride, Pentazocine, Levorphanoltartarate.

   Narcotic Antagonists: Nalorphine hydrochloride, Levallorphantartarate, Naloxone hydrochloride.

   Anti-inflammatory Agents: Sodium salicylate, Aspirin, Mefenamic acid*, Meclofenamate, Indomethacin, Sulindac, Tolmetin, Zomepriac, Diclofenac, Ketorolac, Ibuprofen*, Naproxen, Piroxicam, Phenacetin, Acetaminophen, Antipyrine, Phenylbutazone.

***

Contents

***

INTRODUCTION TO
MEDICINAL CHEMISTRY

♦ LEARNING OBJECTIVES ♦

After completing this unit, reader should be able:

❖ To study definition and importance of medicinal chemistry

❖ To know the history and development of medicinal chemistry

❖ To study various physicochemical properties in relation to biological action

❖ To study various principles of drug metabolism

❖ To learn different factors affecting drug metabolism

Medicinal chemistry is an interdisciplinary field to study combining aspects of organic chemistry, physical chemistry, pharmacology, microbiology, biochemistry as well as computational chemistry. It is concerned with the invention, discovery, design, identification and preparation of biological active compounds, the study of their metabolisms, the interpretation of their mode of action at the molecular level and the construction of "structure-activity relationships".

Medicinal chemistry covers the following stages:

➤ New active substances or drugs are identified and prepared from natural sources, organic chemical reactions or biotechnological processes. They are known as lead molecules.

➤ Optimization of lead structure to improve potency, selectivity and to reduce toxicity.

➤ Development stage, which involves optimization of synthetic route for bulk production and modification of pharmacokinetic and pharmaceutical properties of active substance to render it clinically useful.

During the early stages of medicinal chemistry development, scientists were primarily concerned with the isolation of medicinal agents found in plants. Today, scientists in this field are also equally concerned with the creation of new synthetic compounds as drugs. Medicinal chemistry is almost always geared toward drug discovery and development.

1.1 HISTORY AND DEVELOPMENT OF MEDICINAL CHEMISTRY

The 19th century may be viewed as the birth period of modern medicinal chemistry with the introduction of side chain theory of drug action in 1885 by Berlin immunologist Ehrlich. Later in 1891, he coined the term chemotherapy and defined it as "the chemical entities exhibiting selective toxicities against particular infectious agent. The modern drug receptor theory originated from this side chain theory, which was supported during the same period (mid-1890s) by Cambridge physiologist Langley who described it in his publications as "receptive substances."Research on enzyme specificity (lock-and-key theory) by Fischer in 1894 and Henry's hypothesis on enzyme-substrate complex formation in 1903 are recognized as key advancements in the principles of drug action and modern medicinal chemistry. Grimm's and Erlenmeyer's concepts of isosterism and bioisoterism also had a tremendous impact on the understanding of structure activity relationship (SAR) of drugs and development of modern medicinal chemistry.

Other notable advancements in understanding of drug action and design that were made in the mid to late 20th century include: intervention of charge transfer (Kosower, 1955); induced-fit theory of drug action (Koshland, 1958); concepts of drug latentiation (Harper, 1959) and prodrug (Albert, 1960); application of mathematical methods to medicinal chemistry and transformation of SAR studies into quantitative SAR (QSAR) (Hansch and others, 1960s); and application of artificial intelligence to drug research (Chu, 1974).

Diseases of protozoal and spirochetal origin responded to synthetic chemotherapeutic agents. Interest in synthetic chemicals that could inhibit the rapid reproduction of pathogenic bacteria and enable the host organism to cope with invasive bacteria was dramatically increased when Domagk reported that the red dyestuff 2,4-diaminoazobenzene-4'-sulfonamide (Prontosil) dramatically cured dangerous, systemic gram positive bacterial infections in man and animals. The observation by Woods and Fildes in 1940 that the bacteriostatic action of sulfonamide-like drugs was antagonized by p-aminobenzoic acid, was one of the early examples in which a balance of stimulatory and inhibitory properties depended on the structural analogies of chemicals. Together with the discovery of penicillin by Heming in 1929 and its subsequent examination by Florey and Chain in 1941 led to a water soluble powder of much higher antibacterial potency and lower toxicity than those of previously known synthetic chemotherapeutic agents. With the discovery of a variety of highly potent anti-infective agents, a significant change was introduced into medical practice.

Inventing and developing a new medicine is a long, complex, costly and highly risky process that has few peers in the commercial world. Research and development (R and D) for most of the medicines available today has required 12-24 years for a single new medicine, from starting a project to the launch of a drug product. In addition, many expensive, long-term research projects completely fail to produce a marketable medicine.

In the drug development phase, experience has shown that only approximately about 15-25 drug candidates survive the detailed safety and efficacy testing (in animals and humans) required for it to become a marketed product. Clearly, this is a high-stake, long-term and risky activity, but the potential benefits to the millions of patients with serious diseases provide a constant motivating force.

The most striking differences from the longstanding practice of medicinal chemistry in the new millennium are:

➢ Data reduction of huge amounts of rapidly derived HTS biological results,

➢ Greater emphasis upon multitechnique chemical structure considerations, and most importantly,

➢ The simultaneous attention given to all of the ADMET-related parameters along with efficacy and efficacy-related selectivity (E/S) during lead compound selection and further design or enhancement coupled with an expanding knowledge base that offers the possibility for achieving synergistic benefits by taking advantage of various combinations of multi-agent, prod rug, soft drug, and or multivalent drug strategies.

Medicinal chemists today live in exciting times. They are key participants in the effort to produce more selective, more effective, and safer medicines to treat the diseases of mankind. Their work can have a beneficial effect on millions of suffering patients - surely an important motivating factor for any scientist.

1.2 PHYSICOCHEMICAL PROPERTIES IN RELATION TO BIOLOGICAL ACTION

The ability of a chemical compound to elicit a pharmacological/therapeutic effect is related to the influence of various physical and chemical (*physicochemical*) properties of the chemical substance on the bio molecule that it interacts with.

➢ **Physical Properties:** Physical property of drug is responsible for its action.

➢ **Chemical Properties:** The drug react extracellularly according to simple chemical reactions like neutralization, chelation, oxidation etc.

Various Physico-Chemical Properties are:

❖ Solubility

❖ Partition Coefficient

❖ Ionization

❖ Hydrogen Bonding

❖ Chelation

❖ Surface activity

❖ Isosterism

1.2.1 Solubility

The solubility of a substance at a given temperature is defined as the concentration of the dissolved solute, which is in equillibrium with the solid solute.

Sufficient solubility and membrane permeability is an important factor for oral absorption.

The measurement of aqueous solubility depends upon the following facts.

➢ Buffer and Ionic strength

➢ Polymorphism and Purity of the sample

➢ pH

➢ Super saturation

➢ Thermodynamic versus Kinetic solubility

The solubility of an organic medicinal agents may be expressed in terms of its *affinity/philicity* or *repulsion/phobicity* for either an aqueous (hydro) or lipid (lipo) solvent.

➢ hydrophilic …… water loving.

➢ lipophobic …… lipid hating.

➢ lipophilic …… lipid loving.

➢ hydrophobic …… water hating.

The most important intermolecular attractive forces (bonds) that are involved in the solubilization process are described as follows.

➢ **Vander Waals attraction (induced dipole):** They are weakest intermolecular forces (0.5–1.0 kcal/mole) which occur between nonpolar groups (*e.g.* hydrocarbons). They are highly distance and temperature dependent.

➢ **Dipole-Dipole Bonding:** These forces occur when electronegative elements are attached to carbon. They are stronger (1.0 to 10 kcal/mole) and occur electrostatically between electron deficient and electron rich atoms (dipoles). Hydrogen bonding is a specific example of this bonding and serves as a prime contributor to hydrophilicity.

➢ **Ionic Bonding:** Ionic bond is electrostatic attraction between cations and anions. These ionic attractions are common in inorganic compounds and salts of organic molecules and are relatively strong (5 kcal/mole). Probably the most important factor in the prediction of water solubility in ionic drugs is their ability to ionize. The degree of ionization of a drug is by far the best predictor of solubility for most compounds, which are acidic or basic.

➢ **Ion-Dipole Bonding:** This is electrostatic force between a cation/anion and a dipole. It is relatively strong (1-5 kcal/mole) and is low temperature and distance dependent. Ion dipole bonding is an important attraction between organic medicinal agent and water. Hence, the relative solubility of an organic medicinal agent is a function of the presence of both lipophilic and hydrophilic features within its structure, which serve to determine the extent of interaction of the organic medicinal agent with lipid and/or aqueous phases.

In ascending homologous series, the physico-chemical properties like boiling point, viscosity, surface activity and partition coefficient increase then the aqueous solubility decreases.

The solubility characteristics of a drug can be increased or decreased by derivatisation.

Example: Methyl prednisolone acetate (water insoluble) is changed to Methyl prednisolone sodium succinate (water soluble).

Example: Conversion of chloramphenicol (slightly soluble) to chloramphenicol palmitate (insoluble).

Methods to improve solubility of drugs

➢ Structural modification

➢ Use of cosolvents

➢ Employing surfactants

➢ Complexation

1.2.2 Partition Co-efficient

Partition co-efficient is one of the physico-chemical parameters which influence the drug transport and drug distribution, the way in which the drug reaches the site of action from the site of application.

Partition co-efficient is defined as the equilibrium constant of drug concentration for a molecule in two phases.

- P [Unionized molecule] $= \dfrac{\text{[Drug] lipid}}{\text{[Drug] water}}$

- P [Ionized molecule] $= \dfrac{\text{[Drug] lipid}}{[1 - a][\text{Drug] water}}$

where, a = degree of ionization in aqueous solution.

Factors affecting Partition Co-efficient:

➢ pH

➢ Cosolvents

➢ Surfactant

➢ Complexation

Partition co-efficients are difficult to measure in living system. They are usually determined in vitro 1-octanol as a lipid phase and phosphate buffer of pH 7.4 as the aqueous phase.

The partition co-efficient, P is dimensionless and its logarithm, log P is widely used as the measure of lipophilicity.

The log P is measured by the following methods:

➢ Shake flask method

➢ Chromatographic method

➢ Spectroscopy method

Phenobarbitone has a high lipid/water partition coefficient of 5.9. Thiopentone sodium has a chloroform/water partition coefficient of about 100, so it is highly soluble in lipid.

1.2.3 Surfactant

Surfactant is defined as a material that can reduce the surface tention of water at low concentration. Surface active agents affect the drug absorption which depends on:

➢ The chemical nature of surfactant.

➢ Its concentration.

➢ Its effect on biological membrane and the miscellaneous formation.

At lower concentration the surfactant enhances the absorption rate, the same in higher concentrations reduce the absorption rate.

Applications:

➢ The anthelmentic activity of hexylresorcinol.

➢ Bactericidal activity of cationic quaternary ammonium compounds.

➢ Bactericidal activity of aliphatic alcohols.

➢ Disinfectant action of phenol and cresol.

1.2.4 Hydrogen Bond

The hydrogen bond is a special dipole-dipole interaction between non-bonding electron pairs of hetero atoms like N, S, O and electron deficient hydrogen atom in polar bonds such as OH, NH, F etc.

These are weak bonds and denoted as dotted lines.

$$O-H.......O, \quad HN-H.......O$$

The compounds that are capable of forming hydrogen bonding are only soluble in water. Hydrogen bonding is classified into two types.

Intermolecular Hydrogen Bonding:

In this type, hydrogen bonding occurs between two or more than two molecules of the same compound and results in the formation of polymeric aggregate. Intermolecular hydrogen bonding increases the boiling point of the compound and also its solubility in water. The molecules that are able to develop intermolecular hydrogen bonding improve their solubility by the formation of intermolecular hydrogen bonding with water.

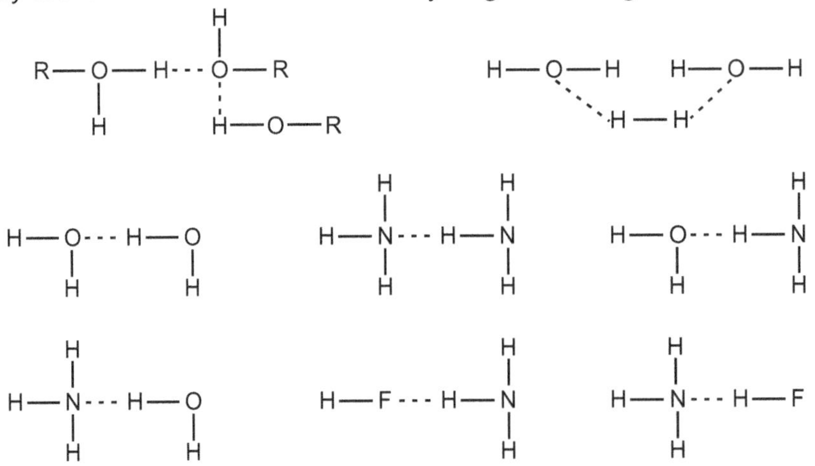

Intramolecular Hydrogen Bonding:

In this type, hydrogen bonding occurs within two atoms of the same molecule. This type of hydrogen bonding is commonly known as chelation and frequently occurs in organic compounds. Sometimes intramolecular hydrogen bonding develops a six or five-membered ring.

Salicylic acid   o-nitrophenol

Hydrogen bonding and biological action

Example: Antipyrin i.e. 1-phenyl 2, 3-dimethyl 5-pyrazolone has analgesic activity.

1-phenyl-3-methyl-5-pyrazolone is inactive

Salicylic acid (o-Hydroxy benzoic acid) has antibacterial activity

para and meta hydroxy benzoic acids are inactive.

1.2.5 Chelation

The compounds that are obtained by donating electrons to a metal ion with the formation of a ring structure are called ***chelates***.

The compounds capable of forming a ring structure with a metal are termed as ***ligands***.

Importance of Chelates in Medicine:

➢ Antidote for metal poisoning.

✓ Dimercaprol is a chelating agent.

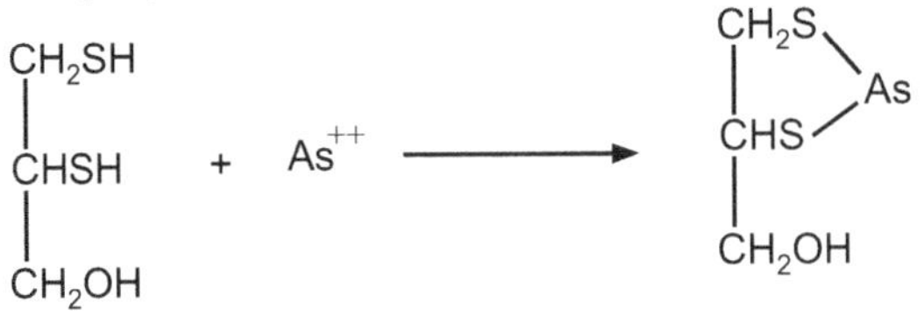

✓ Penicillamine

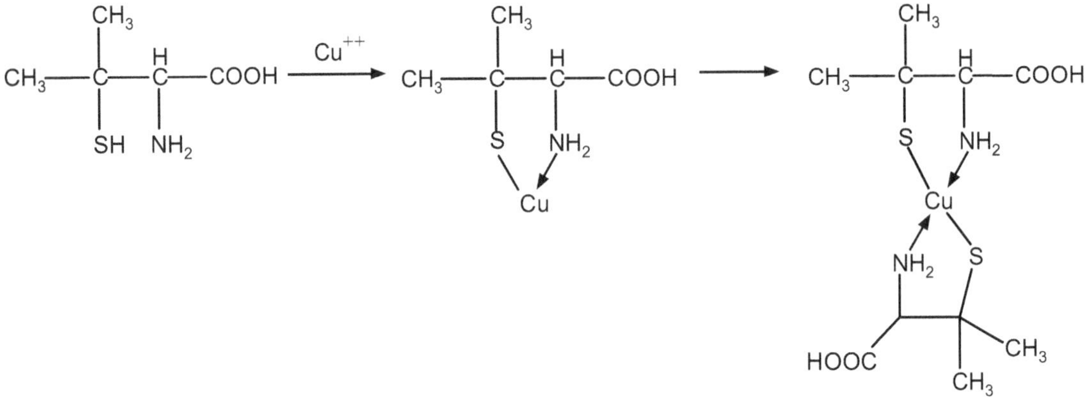

➢ 8-Hydroxyquinoline and its analogs act as antibacterial and anti-fungal agent by complexing with iron or copper.

➢ Undesirable side effects caused by drugs, which chelate with metals.

➢ A side effect of hydralazine-a antihypertensive agent is the formation of anemia and this is due to chelation of the drug with iron.

1.2.6 Ionisation and pK$_a$

Most of the drugs are either weak acids or base and can exist in either ionised or unionised state. The ionisation of the drug depends on its pK$_a$ and pH. The rate of drug absorption is directly proportional to the concentration of the drug at absorbable form but not the concentration of the drug at the absorption site.

o **Example:** Aspirin in stomach will get readily absorbed because it is in the unionised form (99%).

o **Example:** Barbituric acid is inactive because it is strong acid.

5, 5 disubstituted barbituric acid has CNS depressant action because it is a weak acid.

Acids are two types: Unionized acid - HA

Ionized acid - BH$^+$

$$HA + H_2O \rightleftharpoons H_3O^+ + A^-$$

Unionised   Conjugate   Conjugate
acid   acid   base

$$BH^+ \ + \ H_2O \ \rightleftharpoons \ H_3O^+ \ + \ B$$

Ionised   Conjugate   Conjugate
                           acid   base

According to Henderson-Hasselbalch equation,

$$pH = pK_a + \log \frac{[\text{Unionised form}]}{[\text{Ionised form}]}$$

$$\% \text{ ionisation} = \frac{100}{(1 + 10 \, (pH\text{-}pK_a))}$$

By using drug pK_a, the formulation can be adjusted to pH to ensure maximum solubility in water or maximum solubility in non-polar solvent. The pH of a substance can be adjusted to maintain water solubility and complete ionisation.

Example: Phenytoin injection must be adjusted to pH 12 with sodium hydroxide to obtain 99.98% of the drug in ionised form.

Tropicamide eye drops, an anti-cholinergic drug has a pK_a of 5.2 and the drug has to be buffered to pH 4 to obtain more than 90% ionisation.

1.2.7 Optical Isomers

Stereochemistry, enantiomers, symmetry and chirality are impotant concepts in therapeutic and toxic effect of drug. A chiral compound containing one asymmetric centre has two enantiomers. Although each enantiomer has identical chemical and physical properties, they may have different physiological activity like interaction with receptor, metabolism and protein binding. A optical isomer in biological action is due to one isomer being able to achieve a three point attachment with its receptor molecule while its enantiomer would only be able to achieve a two point attachment with the same molecule.

Example: Ephedrine and Psuedoephedrine

The category of drugs where the two isomers have qualitatively similar pharmacological activity but have different quantitative potencies.

MP = 37-39
1 gram 20 ml

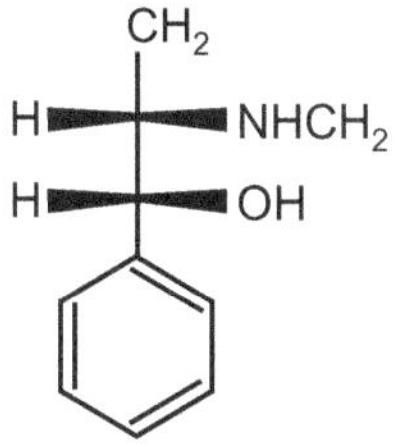

Ephedrine

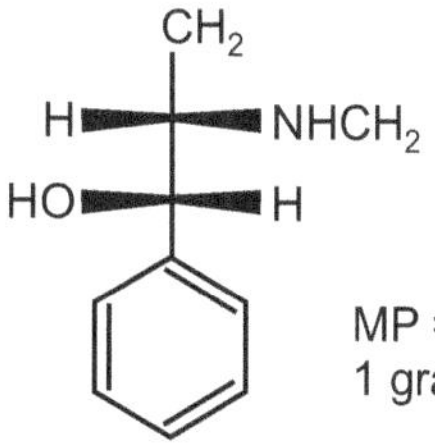

MP = 118-120
1 gram / 200 ml

Pseudoephedrine

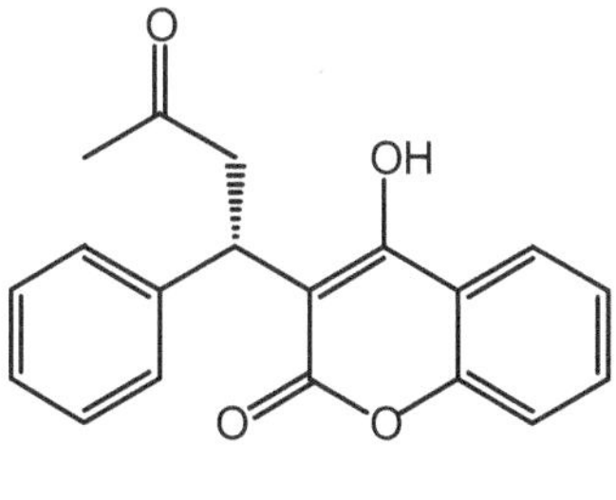

(s)-(−) warfarin

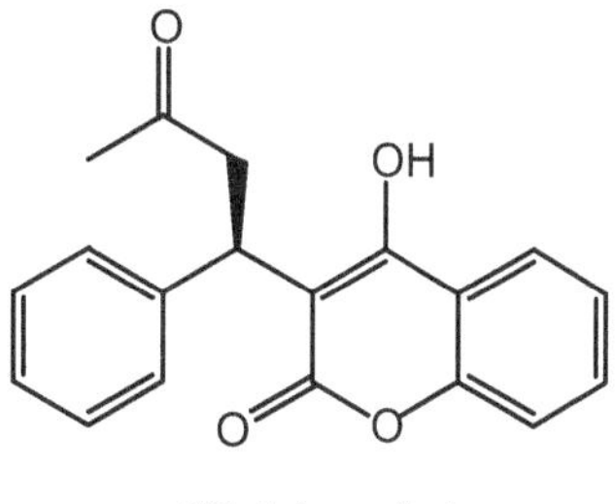

(R)-(+) warfarin

1.2.8 Geometric Isomerism

Geometric isomerism is represented by cis/trans isomerism resulting from restricted rotation due to carbon carbon double bond or in rigid ring system.

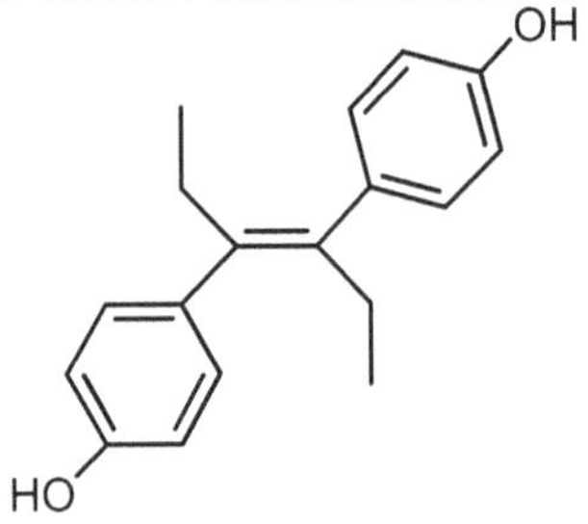

trans-diethylstilbesterol
Estrogenic activity

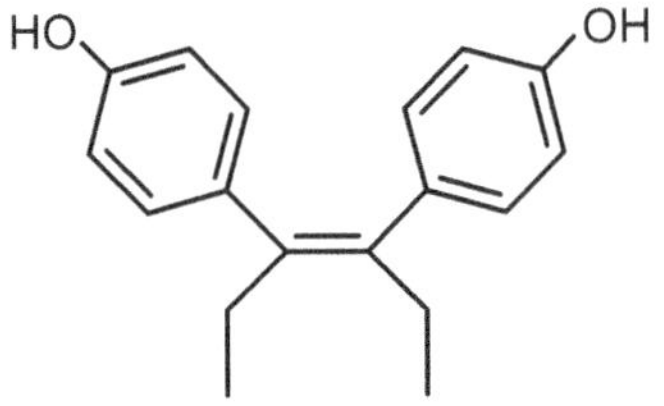

cis-diethylstilbesterol
Only 7% activity
of the trans isomer

1.2.9 Isosterism

Langmuir introduced the term isosterism in 1919, which postulated that two molecules or molecular fragments containing an identical number and arrangement of electron should have similar properties and termed as isosteres. Isosteres should be isoelectric i.e. they should possess same total charge.

Bioisosterism is defined as compounds or groups that possess near or equal molecular shapes and volumes, approximately the same distribution of electron and which exhibit similar physical properties.

They are classified into two types:
➢ Classical bioisosteres
➢ Non-classical bioisosteres.

Classical Bioisosteres:

They have similarities of shape and electronic configuration of atoms, groups and molecules which they replace. The classical bioisosteres may be,

Univalent atoms and groups:
    (i)   Cl, Br, I
    (ii) CH_3NH_2, $-OH$, $-SH$

Bivalent atoms and groups:
    (i)   R-OR, RNH-R, RSR, RSeR
    (ii) $-CONHR$, $-COOR$, $-COSR$

Trivalent atoms and groups:
    (i) $-CH=$, $-N=$
    (ii) $-P=$, $-As=$

Tetravalent atoms and groups:

  $=C=$, $=N=$, $=P=$

Application of Classical Bioisosteres in drug design:

➢ Replacement of $-NH_2$ group by $-CH_3$ group.

Carbutamide: R = NH_2

Tolbutamide: R = CH_3

$$R-\langle\!\bigcirc\!\rangle-SO_2NH\ CONH(CH_2)_3CH_3$$

➢ Replacement of $-OH$ and $-SH$

Guanine = $-OH$

6-Thioguanine = $-SH$

Non-classical Bioisosteres:

They do not obey the stearic and electronic definition of classical isosteres. These isosteres retain activity by the retention of their properties such as pK_a, electrostatic potentials, which can alter selective enzyme processes.

Examples:

- Halogens: Cl, F, Br,CN
- Ether: -S-, -O-
- Carbonyl group

- Hydroxyl group $-OH$, $-NHSO_2R$, CH_2OH
- Catechol

Catechol

1.2.10 Protein Binding

The reversible binding of protein with non-specific and non-functional site on the body protein without showing any biological effect is called as protein binding.

$$\text{Protein + Drug} \rightleftharpoons \text{Protein-drug complex}$$

Depending on the whether the drug is a weak or strong acid, base or is neutral, it can bind to single blood proteins to multiple proteins. The most significant protein involved in the binding of drug is albumin, which comprises more than half of blood volume.

1.3 METABOLISM

Metabolism is the body's mechanism for processing, using, inactivating, and eventually eliminating foreign substances, including drugs. Drug exerts its influence upon the body, it is gradually metabolized, or neutralized. The liver, the blood, the lymph fluid, or any body tissue that recognizes the drug as a foreign substance can break down or alter the chemical structure of drugs, making them less active, or inert. Drugs also can be neutralized by diverting them to body fat or proteins, which hold the substances to prevent them from acting on body organs. Once a drug is metabolized, it is the kidneys that normally filter the neutralized particles, called metabolites, as well as other waste and water, from the blood. Drugs can also be excreted out of the body by the lungs, in sweat, or in feces.

Metabolism is an essential pharmacokinetic process, which renders lipid soluble and non-polar compounds to water soluble and polar compounds so that they are excreted by various processes. This is because only water-soluble substances undergo excretion, whereas lipid soluble substances are passively reabsorbed from renal or extra renal excretory sites into the blood by virtue of their lipophilicity. Metabolism is a necessary biological process that limits the life of a substance in the body.

1.4 SITE OF DRUG METABOLISM

The major site of drug metabolism is the liver (microsomal enzyme systems of hepatocytes). The primary site for metabolism of almost all drugs because it is relatively rich in a large variety of metabolising enzymes. Secondary organs of biotransformation; Kidney (proximal tubule), Lungs (Type II cells), Testes (Sertoli cells), Skin (epithelial cells), plasma, nervous tissue (brain), intestines. Metabolism by organs other than liver (called as extra-hepatic metabolism) is of lesser importance because lower level of metabolising enzymes is present in such tissues. Within a cell, drug metabolising activity is found in the smooth endoplasmic reticulum (microsomes) and the cytosol. Drug metabolism can also occur in mitochondria, nuclear envelope and plasma membrane.

A few drugs are also metabolised by non-enzymatic means called as non-enzymatic metabolism. e.g. atracurium, a neuromuscular blocking drug, is inactivated in plasma by spontaneous non-enzymatic degradation (Hoffman elimination) in addition to that by pseudocholinesterase enzyme.

1.5 METABOLIC REACTION OR BIOTRANSFORMATION REACTIONS

Metabolic conversions are classified as either Phase-I (oxidation, reduction or hydrolysis), or Phase II (conjugation). The enzymes involved in Phase-I reactions are primarily located in the endoplasmic reticulum of the liver cell, they are called microsomal enzymes. Phase-I reactions are non-synthetic in nature, and generally produce more water soluble and less active metabolite. The most common phase-I reactions are:

- Oxidative processes (aromatic hydroxylation; aliphatic hydroxylation; N-, O-, and S-dealkylation; N-hydroxylation; N-oxidation; sulfoxidation; deamination; and dehalogenation).

- Reductive process (azodye-reduction, nitroreduction) and
- Hydrolytic reactions.

Phase-I reactions	**Phase-II reactions (Conjugations)**
1. Oxidation 2. Reduction 3. Hydrolysis	1. Glucuronidation 2. Sulfation 3. Conjugation with glycine (Gly) 4. Conjugation with glutathione (GSH) 5. Acetylation 6. Methylation

1.6 PHASE-I REACTION

Oxidation:

It is an important metabolic reaction. Energy is derived by oxidative combustion of organic compounds containing carbon and hydrogen atoms. During oxidation reaction, the hydrophilicity of drugs were increased by addition of functional group. Enzymes involved in the phase-I oxidative reaction are microsomal mono-oxygenases or mixed functional oxidases (MAO). These reactions require molecular oxygen (O_2) and reducing $NADPH^+H^+$ for the reaction which were located in the endoplasmic reticulum of liver.

Oxidation	
Microsomal catalysed by	**Non-microsomal catalysed by:**
• Cytochrome P-450 (CYP)	• Monoamino-oxidases (MAO) - mitochondrial.
• Microsomal flavine-containing monooxigenase (FMO).	• Mo-containing oxidases (cytosolic): Xanthine oxidase (XO) and Aldehyde oxidase (AOX).
	• Alcohol and aldehyde dehydrogenases (ADH, ALDH) cytosolic.

Oxidations Catalyzed by Cytochrome P-450 (CYP):

CYP is a heme-containing protein embedded in the membranes of the smooth endoplasmic reticulum (SER), the fragments of which in a tissue homogenate are sedimented after ultracentrifugation (at 100,000 g) in the microsomal fraction.

CYP constitutes a super family of enzymes that are classified into families (numbered) and subfamilies (marked with capital letters), the latter of which contain the individual enzymes (numbered), e.g., CYP1A2, CYP2C9, CYP2D6, CYP3A4.

CYP is an extremely versatile enzyme as it can catalyze numerous types of reaction, out of which three types are presented below.

Oxygenation:

Oxygenation involves insertion of an O atom (from O_2) into a C-H bond, forming a hydroxylated metabolite, or into a C=C double bond, forming an epoxide. A hydroxylated metabolite may be stable, or unstable. From an unstable hydroxylated metabolite, a group may break off spontaneously: an alkyl group, ammonia, a halogen atom, or sulfur atom; such reactions are called oxidative dealkylation, oxidative deamination, oxidative dehalogenation, and oxidative desulfuration, respectively.

General scheme:

$$RH + O_2 + (NADPH + H)^+ \xrightarrow[\text{NADPH-CYP reductase}]{\text{CYP}} R - OH + HOH + NADP^+$$

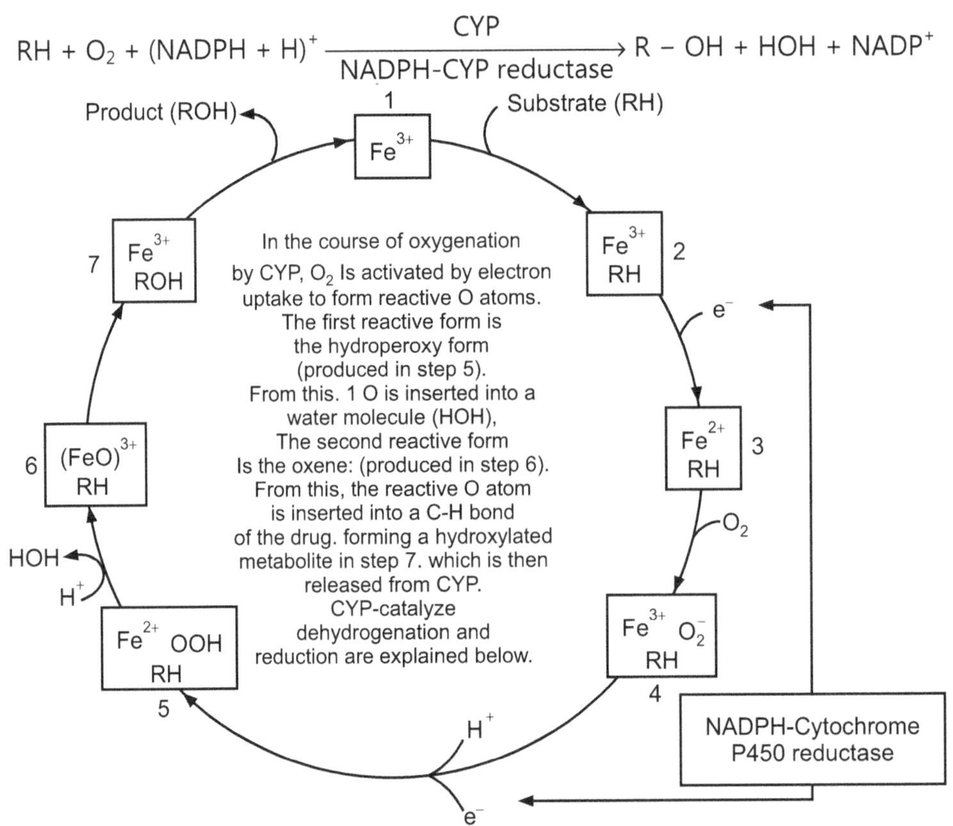

Note: that Fe represents the iron in CYP.

Insertion of it produces a Stable Metabolite (Oxygenation):

(a) Hydroxylation:

- ➤ **C-hydroxylation** (insertion of *O into a C−H bond to form a hydroxyl group*).

    - Aliphatic hydroxylation: Tolbutamide (−), terfenadine (+), cyclophosphamide (+).

    - Aromatic hydroxylation: Warfarin (−), phenytoin (−), propranolol (−).

- ➤ **N-hydroxylation** (insertion of *O into an N-H bond*): dapsone.

C-hydroxylation: Aliphatic:

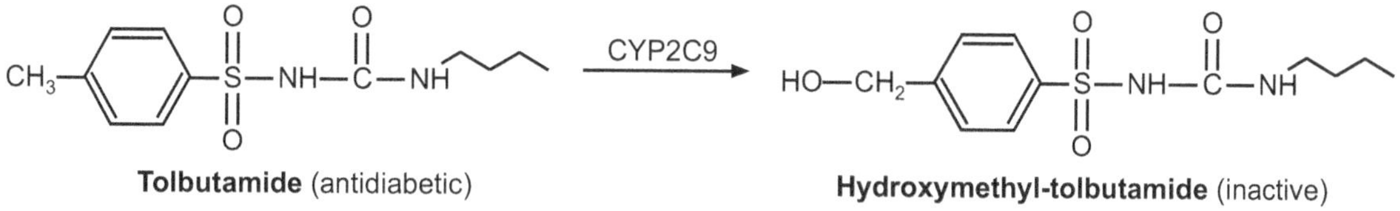

Tolbutamide (antidiabetic)

CYP2C9

Hydroxymethyl-tolbutamide (inactive)

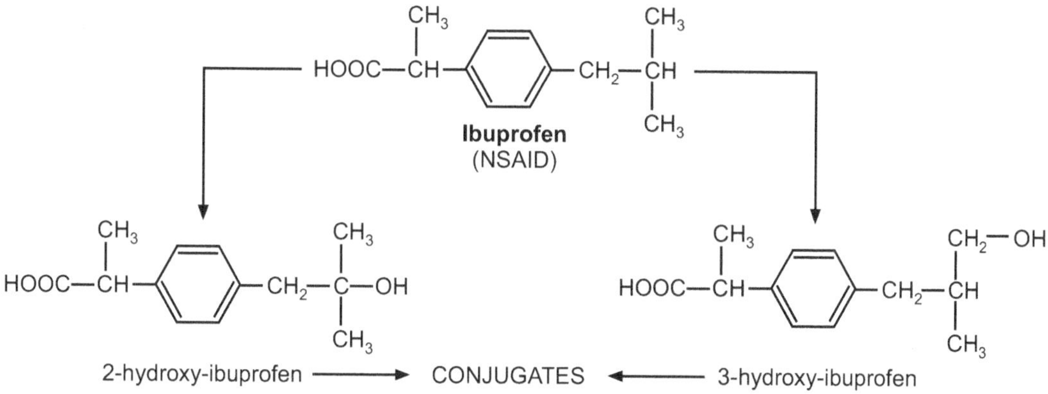

Ibuprofen
(NSAID)

2-hydroxy-ibuprofen ⟶ CONJUGATES ⟵ 3-hydroxy-ibuprofen

C-hydroxylation: Aromatic:

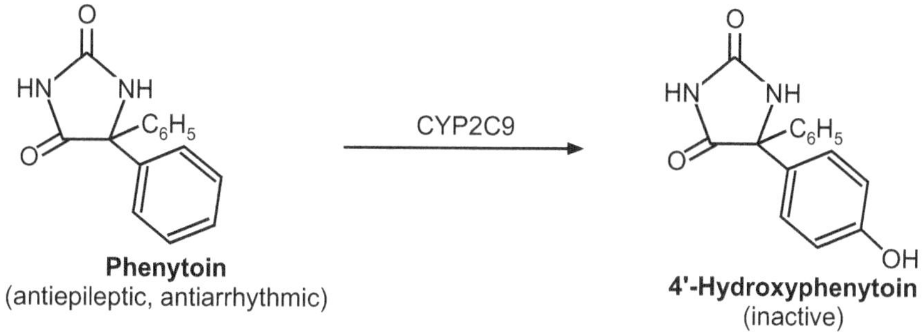

Phenytoin
(antiepileptic, antiarrhythmic)

CYP2C9

4'-Hydroxyphenytoin
(inactive)

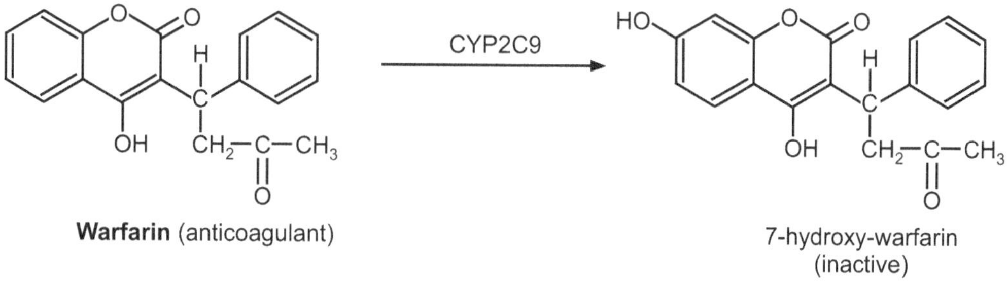

Warfarin (anticoagulant)

CYP2C9

7-hydroxy-warfarin
(inactive)

N-hydroxylation:

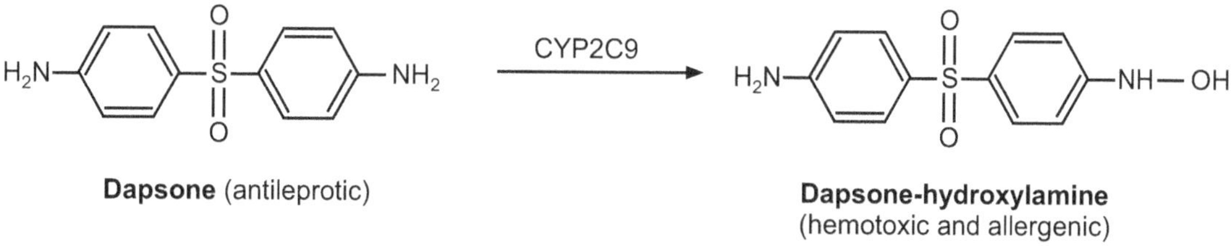

Dapsone (antileprotic)

CYP2C9

Dapsone-hydroxylamine
(hemotoxic and allergenic)

(b) Epoxidation (insertion of *O into a C = C bond to form an epoxide*): Carbamazepine.

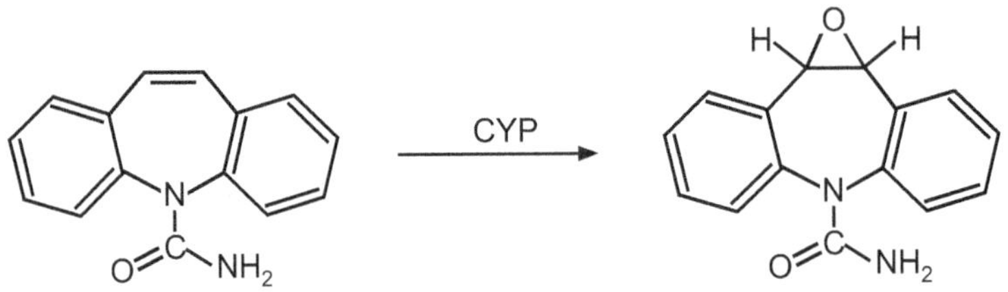

CYP

Carbamazepine
(antiepileptic)

Carbamazepine-10,11-epoxide
(less active metabolite)

Insertion of it produces an Unstable Metabolite (Oxygenation):

First, the drug becomes hydroxylated at the C atom of the alkyl group that is linked to the N (or the O) atom. This hydroxylated metabolite is unstable. It breaks spontaneously into two molecules: the dealkylated metabolite (e.g., an amine or alcohol/phenol), and an aldehyde (e.g., formaldehyde after demethylation, acetaldehyde after deethylation, etc.).

Oxidative dealkylation (dealkylated metabolite + *an aldehyde*):

(a) N-dealkylation: Diazepam → nordiazepam (+), Carisoprodol → meprobamate (+), Amitriptyline → nortriptyline (+) → desmethyl-nortriptyline (−) Lidocaine → monoethylglycylxylidine (+) → glycylxylidine (−) Caffeine → paraxanthine (−), or theophylline, or theobromine.

N-dealkylation: Example:

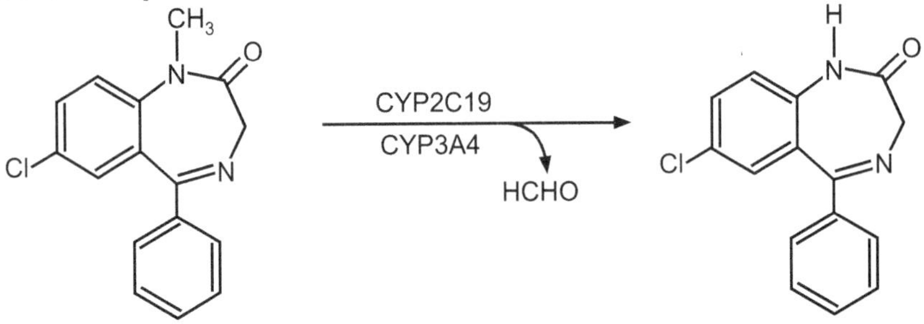

CYP2C19
CYP3A4
HCHO

Diazepam

Nordiazepam

O-dealkylation: Example:

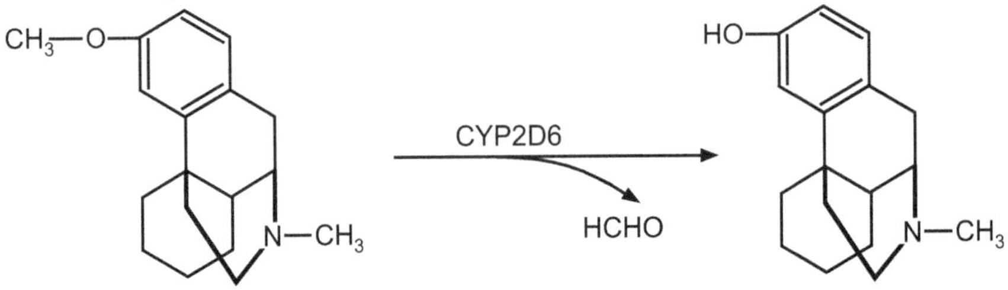

CYP2D6
HCHO

Dextromethorphan
(antitussive drug)

Dextrorphan
(active metabolite)

(b) Oxidative deamination ($\rightarrow$ O-containing metabolite + NH_3):

Amphetamine $\rightarrow$ Phenylacetone ($-$)

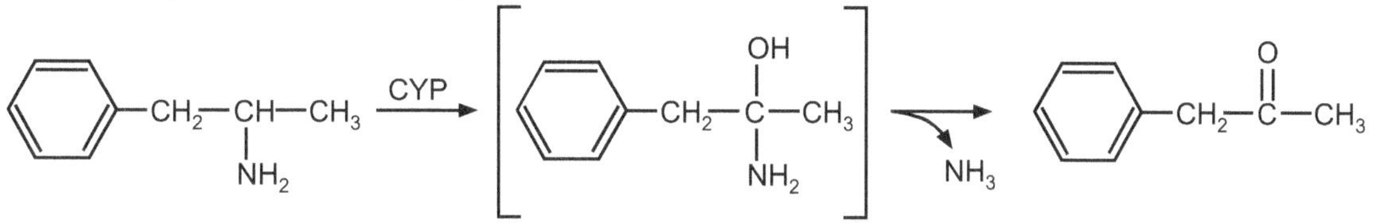

Amphetamine
(centrally acting sympathomimetic)

Phenyl acetone
(inactive)

(c) Oxidative dehalogenation ($\rightarrow$ O-containing metabolite + HBr):

Halothane $\rightarrow$ trifluoroacetyl chloride (+)

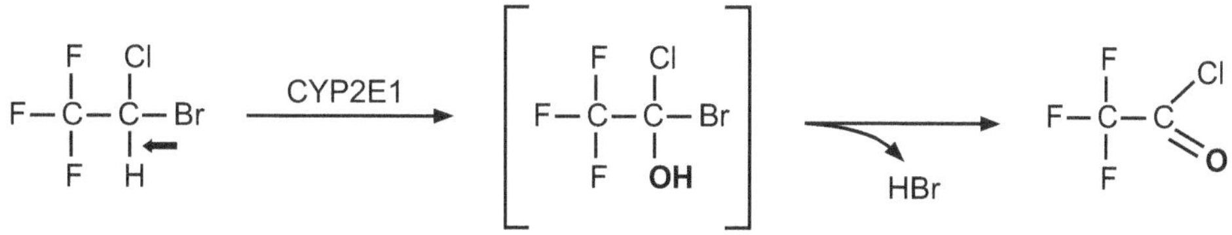

Halothane
(inhalation anesthetic)

Trifluoro-acetyl-chloride

(d) Oxidative desulfuration ($\rightarrow$ O-containing metabolite + S):

Thiopenthal $\rightarrow$ Pentobarbital (+), Parathion $\rightarrow$ Paraoxon (+)

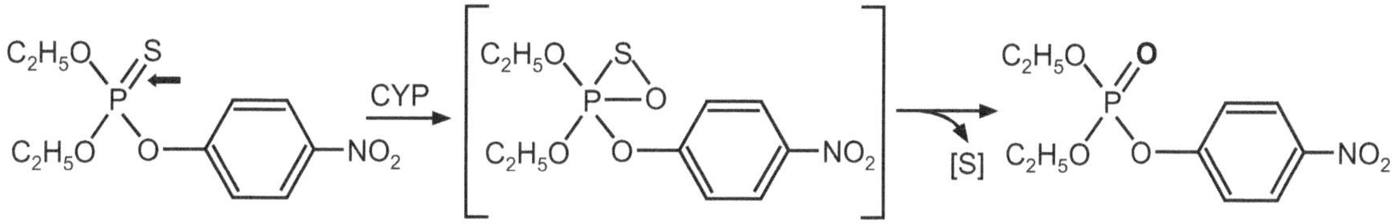

Parathion
(an organophosphate insecticide)

Paraoxon
(active insecticide,
an irreversible inhibitor of
acetylcholinesterase)

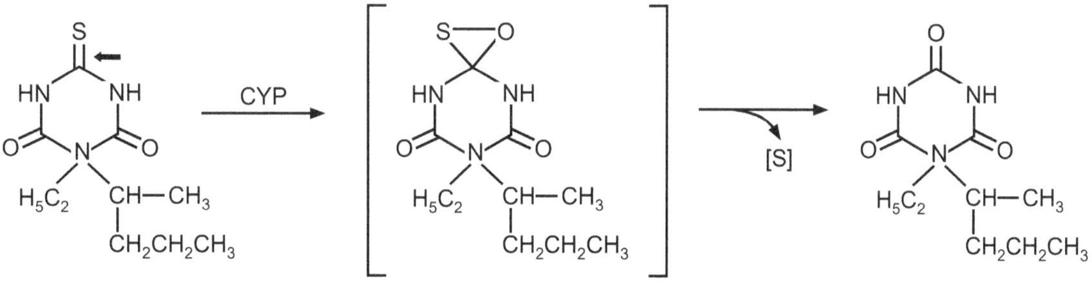

Thiopental

Pentobarbital

CYP-Catalyzed Dehydrogenation Reactions:

CYP also catalyze **dehydrogenation**, i.e. removal of 2 H atoms from a drug molecule (this is how the reactive hepatotoxic paracetamol metabolite is formed).

General scheme:

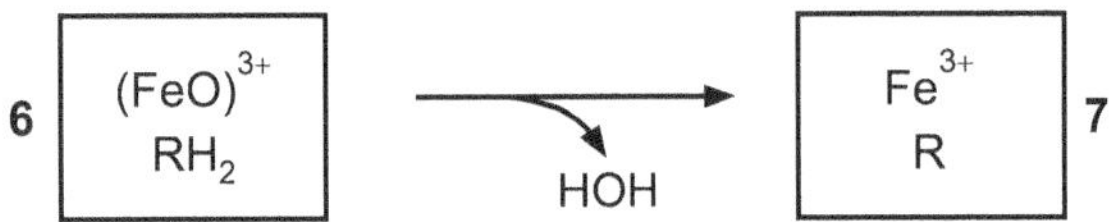

NOTE: While an oxygenation produces 1 molecule hydroxylated metabolite plus 1 molecule HOH, dehydrogenation produces 2 molecules HOH.

Note: While an oxygenation produces 1 molecule hydroxylated metabolite plus 1 molecule HOH, dehydrogenation produces 2 molecules HOH.

Examples:

Acetaminophen
analgetic and
antipyretic drug

N-Acetyl-p-benzo-quinoneimine
(NAPBQI)
hepatotoxic

Nifedipine

"Pyridine metabolite"

S-dealkylation: S-dealkylation involves oxidative cleavage of alkyl carbon-sulfur bonds.

6-(Methylthio)-purine　　　　　Hydroxylated intermediate　　　　　6-Mercaptopurine

Desulfuration:

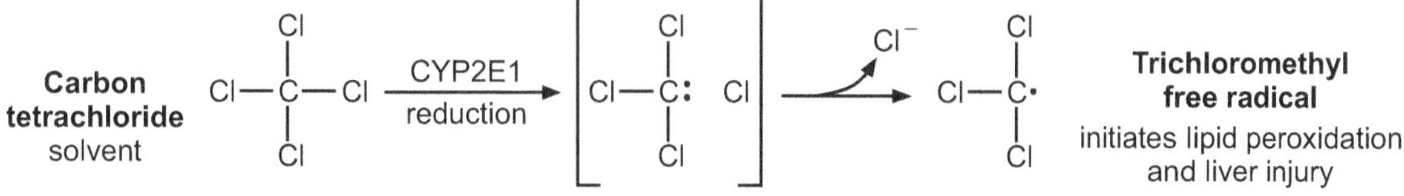

Thiopental
(an i,v. anesthetic)

Pentobarbital
(active as hypnotic)

CYP-catalyzed Reduction Reactions:

CYP may also catalyze reduction, by transferring only 1 electron to a compound (e.g. in a reductive dehalogenation reaction) or as many as 6 electrons to a nitro group, thus converting it into an amino group (nitro reduction). In CYP-catalyzed reduction, the second electron is not transferred to the CYP-bound O_2, but to the CYP-bound substrate, e.g. carbon tetrachloride or clonazepam (see also under nitro reduction). With carbon tetrachloride, its reduced intermediate then undergoes a homolytic cleavage to form a free radical and a chloride anion. The reactive trichloromethyl free radical formed in the liver, can initiate lipid peroxidation in the liver cell membranes and can thus induce hepatic necrosis.

General Scheme:

Reductive dehalogenation of carbon tetrachloride (1-electron reduction):

Nitro-reduction of clonazepam to 7-amino-clonazepam (6-electron reduction):

Clonazepam
anxiolytic and
antiepileptic drug

7-amino-clonazepam
inactive

Oxidations catalyzed by Microsomal Flavin-containing Monooxygenase (FMO):

- Oxidation of S atom: Cimetidine → cimetidine-S-oxide.

- Oxidation of tert. N atom: Nicotine → nicotine-1-N-oxide, Trimethylamine → trimethylamine N-oxide.

S-oxidation:

Cimetidine
(an H_2-receptor antagonist)

Cimetidine S-oxide
(inactive)

N-oxidation:

Nicotine

Nicotine-1'-N -oxide
(inactive)

Trimethylamine

Trimethylamine N-oxide

Oxidations catalyzed by non-microsomal enzymes:

The oxygen incorporated into the substrate is derived from HOH rather than O_2.

- MAO catalyzes oxidative deamination of amines:

Examples: Dopamine → 3,4-dihydroxy-phenylacetaldehyde.

Norepinephrine → 3,4-dihydroxy-mandelic aldehyde (−).

Four Steps: The byproducts are ammonia and HOOH

1. $R - CH_2NH_2 + FAD > R - CH = NH + FADH_2$ Dehydrogenation
2. $R - CH = NH + H_2O > R - CH(OH) - NH_2$ Hydration
3. $R - CH(OH) - NH_2 > R - CH = O + NH_2$ Deamination
4. $FADH_2 + O_2 > FAD + H_2O_2$ FAD

3,4-dihydroxy-
phenyl acetyl aldehyde
(DOPAL)

Acid (DOPAC)

Oxidation by ALDH
Reduction by AR

Alcohol

- **Xanthine oxidase-catalyzed oxidation:**

  Examples: Hypoxanthine → Xanthine → Uric acid

  Allopurinol → Alloxanthine

  Hypoxanthine   **Xanthine**   **Uric acid**

- **Aldehyde oxidase-catalyzed oxidation:**

  Examples: Nicotine → 1′(5′) iminium ion → Cotinine - Benzaldehyde → Benzoic acid

oxidation.

Nicotine

CYP2A6
CYP2B6
Dehydrogenation

Nicotine-$\Delta^{1'(5)}$-iminium ion

AOX
HOH

O_2 / AOX
HOOH

Cotinine

Benzaldehyde

AOX
HOH

AOX
O_2 / HOOH

Benzoic acid

- **Oxidations catalyzed by alcohol and aldehyde dehydrogenases:**

   Examples: Methanol → Formaldehyde → Formic acid

   Ethanol → Acetaldehyde → Acetic acid.

$CH_3 - CH_2 - OH$ NAD^+ $NADH + H^+$ **ADH** → $CH_3 - C(=O)H$ HOH → $[CH_3 - C(OH)(H)(OH)]$ NAD^+ $NADH + H^+$ **ALDH** → $CH_3 - C(=O)OH$

Ethanol   **Acetaldehyde**   **Acetic acid**

DISULFIRAM
to promote
alcohol withdrawal

$CH_3 - OH$ NAD^+ $NADH + H^+$ **ADH** → $H - C(=O)H$ HOH → $[H - C(OH)(H)(OH)]$ NAD^+ $NADH + H^+$ **ALDH** → $H - C(=O)OH$

Methanol   **Formaldehyde**   **Formic acid**

ETHANOL
FOMEPIZOLE
(antidotes)

Formic acid causes acidosis
and retinal injury (blindness)

Reduction:

- **Azo-reduction - catalyzed by *microbial enzymes* in the colon.**

   Example: Prontosyl → Sulfanilamide + Triaminobenzene,

   Sulfasalazine (salicylazosulfapyridine) → 5-aminosalicylic acid sulfapyridine.

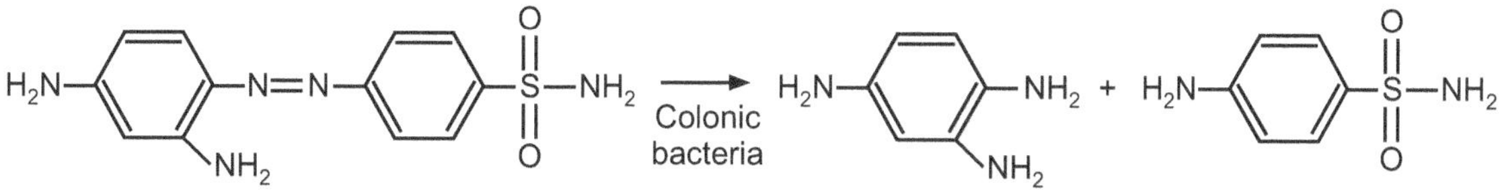

Prontosil   **Triaminobenzene**   **Sulfanilamide**

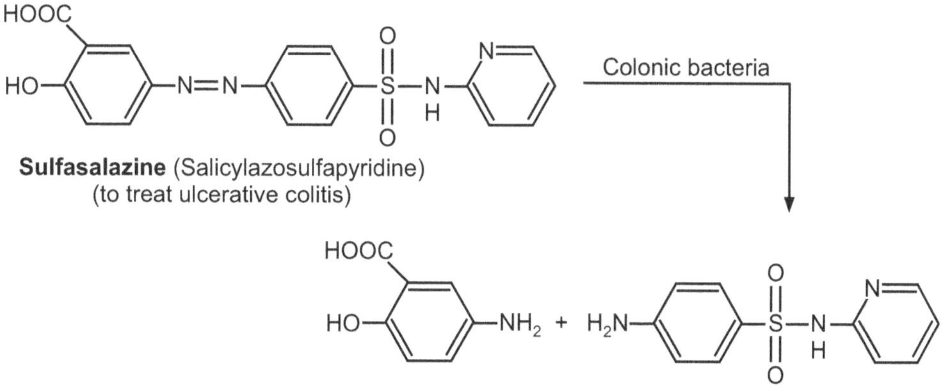

Colonic bacteria

Sulfasalazine (Salicylazosulfapyridine)
(to treat ulcerative colitis)

Colonic bacteria

5-amInosalicylic acid
(antiinflammatory)

Sulfapyridine

- **Nitro-reduction catalyzed by CYP**

  Example: Clonazepam $\rightarrow$ 7-amino-clonazepam.

  Chloramphenicol $\rightarrow$ An arylamine metabolite.

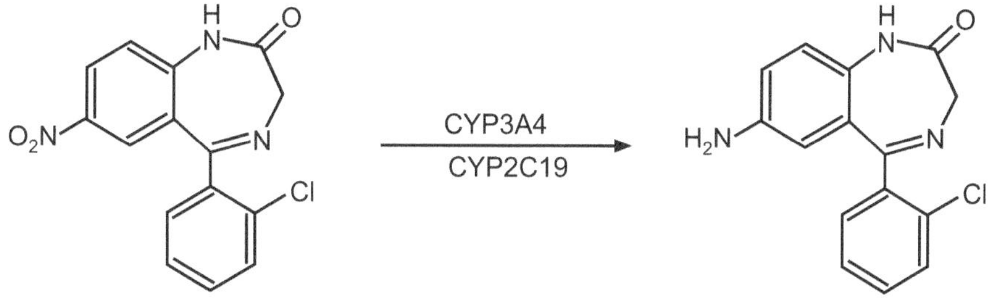

CYP3A4
CYP2C19

Clonazepam
(anxiolytic and
antiepileptic effects)

7-amino-clonazepam
(inactive)

Hydrolysis:

Hydrolysis of esters: The active drugs are converted into inactive (or less active) metabolites. E.g. Succinylcholine, procaine, meperidine, acetylsalicylic acid.

By alkaline phosphatases: hydrolyzes phosphoric acid monoesters

Examples: (i.v. injectable prodrugs): Phosphenytoin (−) Phenytoin (+) Phospropofol (−) Propofol (+) Clindamycin phosphate (−) Clindamycin (+).

Phosphenytoin

Phenytoin

Phospropofol

Propofol

Hydrolysis by Paraoxonases (PON):

➢ **Hydrolysis of phosphoric acid tri-esters**

Examples: Paraoxon and other organophosphate insecticides.

Paraoxon

➢ **Hydrolysis of lactones:**

Examples: Statins, e.g. lovastatin, or simvastatin (lactone) → Hydroxy-acid (+),
Spironolactone → Hydroxy-acid (−)

Lovastatin
(HMG-CoA reductase inhibitor,
cholesterol lowering drug)

Spironolactone
(aldosterone antagonist, K-sparing diuretic)

1.7 PHASE-II REACTIONS (CONJUGATIONS)

Phase-II reactions were also as conjugation reactions. Metabolic transformation of drugs in phase-I generally produced less water souble or pharmacologically inactive metabolites. Some exhibit more or less or different activity from the parent drug. Phase-II reactions or conjugation as glucoronic acid, sulphate, acetyl group or other amino acids in presence of enzyme transferasesand then excreted out.

Phase-II reactions (conjugations) involved the following reactions:

- ➢ Glucuronidation.
- ➢ Sulfation.
- ➢ Conjugation with glycine (Gly), glutamine and other amino acids.
- ➢ Conjugation with glutathione (GSH) or mercaptopuric acid.
- ➢ Acetylation.
- ➢ Methylation.

Glucuronidation:

Glucuronidation involves the reaction of drug metabolite with glucuronic acid in presence of enzyme UDP-glucuronyl transferase. Drug substrate attached to glucuronic acid of uridine diphosphate glucuronic acid (UDPGA). Glucuronides thus formed are inactive and excreted into the urine and bile. Molecules with phenolic hydroxyl, alcoholic hydroxyl, and carboxylic acid groups undergo glucuronidation reaction readily.

Glu-1-P → UDPG → UDPGA → Substrate drug molecule → Glucuronide metabolites.

Structure of UDPGA:

Ether glucuronide formation (from compounds with a hydroxyl group).

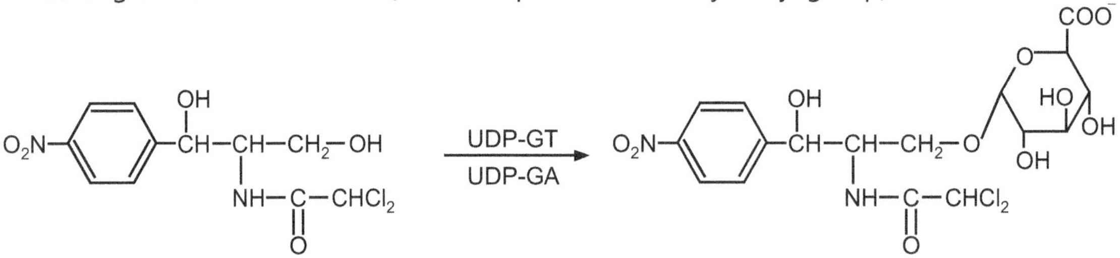

Chloramphenicol
(antibiotic)

Chloramphenicol glucuronide
(rapidly excreted in urine)

Ester glucuronide formation (from compounds with a carboxylic group).

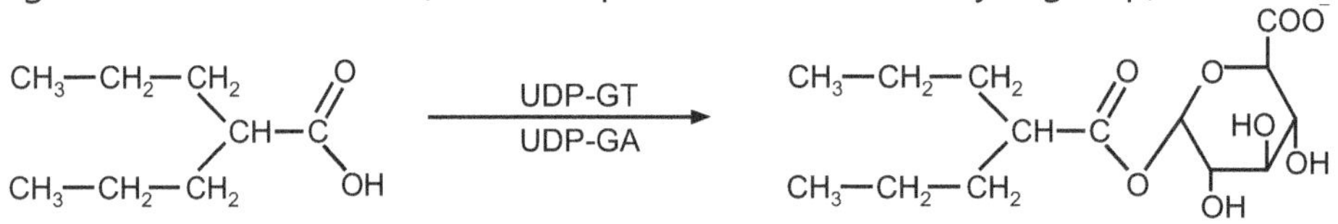

Valproic acid
(antiepileptic drug)

Valproic acid glucuronide
(rapidly excreted in urine)

Sulfation:

Sulfation sulphate conjugates are formed by the conjugation of sulphate moiety with the drug substrate. Compounds containing alcoholic hydroxyl, phenolic hydroxyl and other compounds containing amino group undergo sulphate conjugation. The sulphate moiety from cofactor 3'-phosphoadenosine-5'-phosphosulphate (PAPS). The transfer of sulphate takes place in the presence of enzyme sulphotransferase.

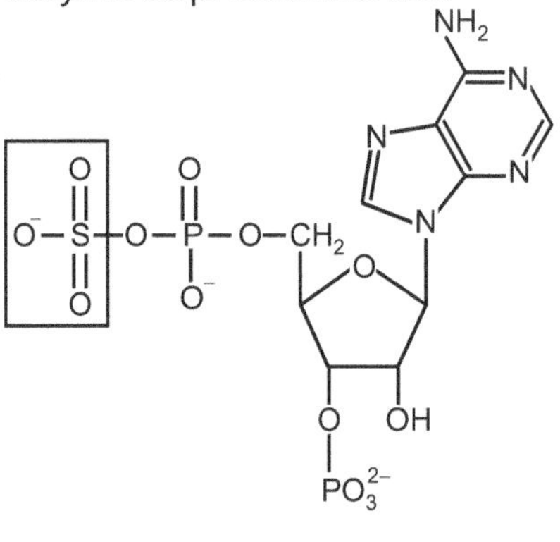

Examples:

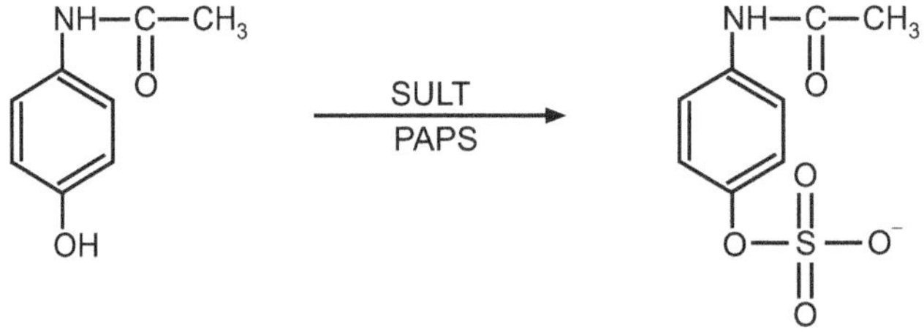

Acetaminophen = paracetamol
(analgetic and antipyretic)

Acetaminophen-sulfate = paracetamol-sulfate
(rapidly excreted in urine)

Conjugation with Glycine (GLY)

Examples:

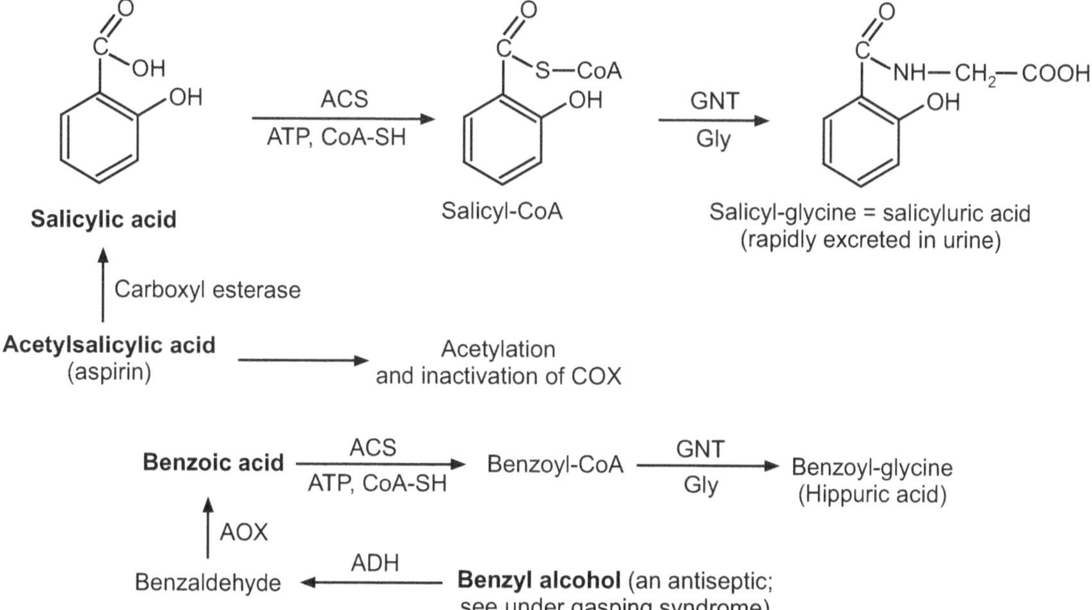

Salicylic acid → (ACS, ATP, CoA-SH) → Salicyl-CoA → (GNT, Gly) → Salicyl-glycine = salicyluric acid (rapidly excreted in urine)

Acetylsalicylic acid (aspirin) — Carboxyl esterase → Salicylic acid

Acetylsalicylic acid (aspirin) → Acetylation and inactivation of COX

Benzoic acid → (ACS, ATP, CoA-SH) → Benzoyl-CoA → (GNT, Gly) → Benzoyl-glycine (Hippuric acid)

Benzaldehyde → (AOX) → **Benzoic acid**

Benzyl alcohol (an antiseptic; see under gasping syndrome) → (ADH) → Benzaldehyde

Conjugation with Glutathione (GSH) or Mercaptopuric Acid:

Enzymes: Glutathione S-transferases (GST).

Cosubstrate: Glutathione (GSH).

γ-glutamic acid   Cysteine   Glycine

Acetaminophen = Paracetamol → (CYP2E1, Toxication) → **N-acetyl-p-benzo-quinoneimine (NAPBQI)** → (GSH, Detoxication) → Acetaminophen-glutathione conjugate (readily excreted)

ELECTROPHILIC METABOLITE
MAY CAUSE HEPATIC NECROSIS

Acetylation:

Enzymes: N-acetyltransferases (NAT).

Cosubstrate: Acetyl coenzyme A (Ac-CoA).

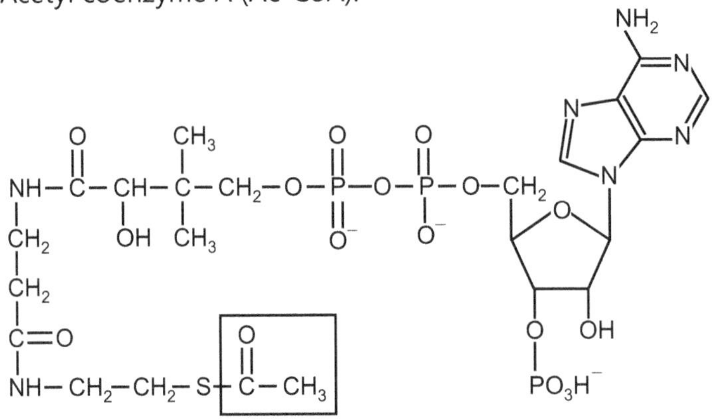

Examples:

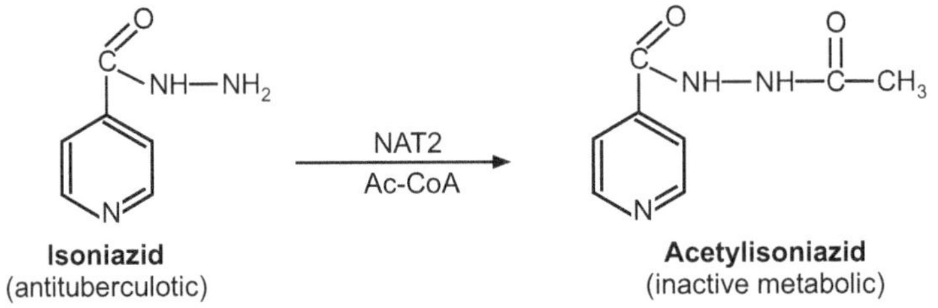

Isoniazid
(antituberculotic)

NAT2
Ac-CoA

Acetylisoniazid
(inactive metabolic)

Methylation:

Enzymes: Methyltransferases (MT).

Cosubstrate: S-aldenocylmethionine (SAM).

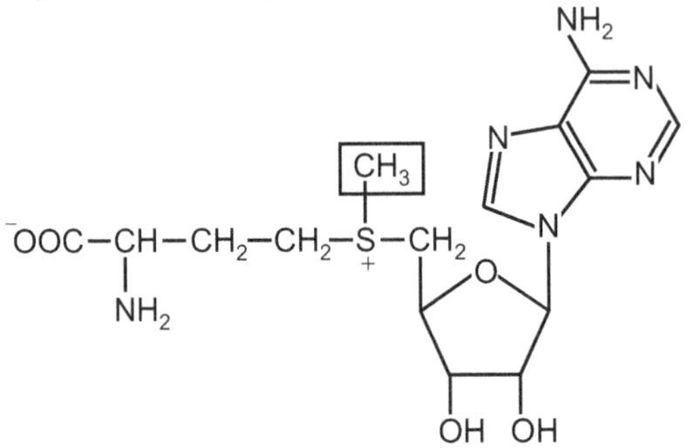

Example:

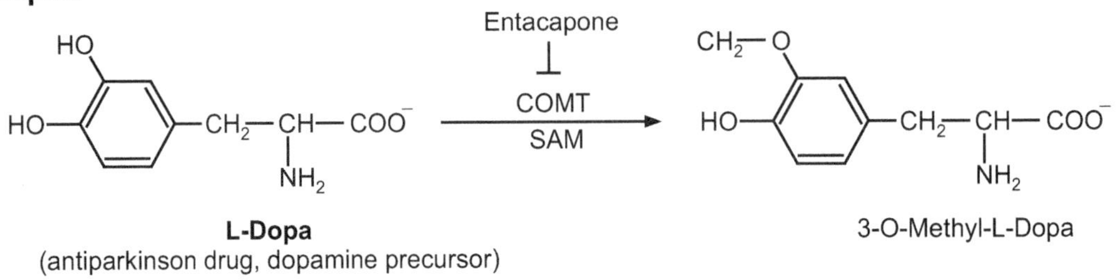

Entacapone

COMT
SAM

L-Dopa
(antiparkinson drug, dopamine precursor)

3-O-Methyl-L-Dopa

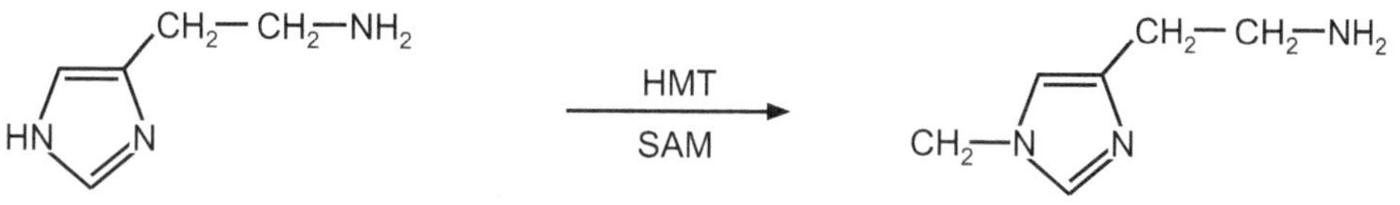

Histamine → (HMT / SAM) → **N-Methylhistamine**

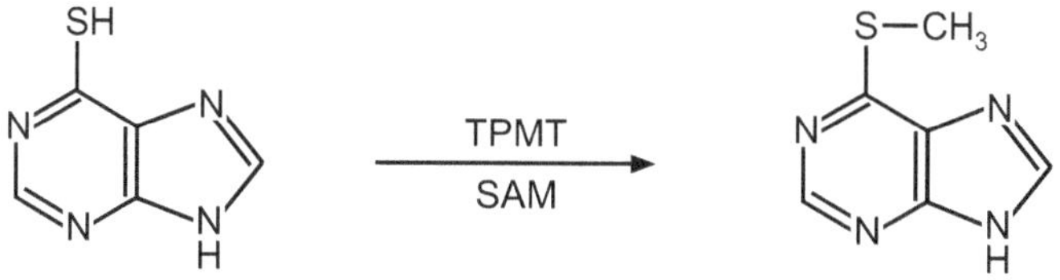

6-Mercaptopurine
(antitumor drug) → (TPMT / SAM) → **6-Methylmercaptopurine**

Factors affecting drug metabolism including stereo chemical aspects:

The therapeutic efficacy, toxicity and biological half-life of a drug greatly depends on the metabolism of the drug and a number of factors affect the metabolism of the drug. Hence various factors affecting drug metabolism must be considered during administration and also in proper dosing of any drug to the patients.

Factors Affecting Metabolism: A number of factors may influence the metabolic rate of a drug. Some of them are:

- Chemical factors which include:
  - (a) Enzyme induction
  - (b) Enzyme inhibition
  - (c) Environmental chemicals
- Biological factors which include:
  - (a) Age
  - (b) Diet
  - (c) Sex difference
  - (d) Species difference
  - (e) Strain difference
  - (f) Altered physiological factors
- Physicochemical properties of the drug

Chemical Factors:

(a) Enzyme induction: The phenomenon of increased drug metabolizing ability of enzymes by several drugs and chemicals is called as enzyme induction and the agents which bring about such an effect are called enzyme inducers.

Mechanisms of enzyme induction:

- Increase in both liver size and liver blood flow.
- Increase in both total and microsomal protein content.
- Increased stability of enzymes.

- Increased stability of cytochrome P-450.
- Decreased degradation of cytochrome P-450.
- Proliferation of smooth endoplasmic reticulum.

Consequences of enzyme induction include:

- Decrease in pharmacological activity of drugs.
- Increased activity where the metabolites are active.
- Altered physiological status due to enhanced metabolism of endogenous compounds such as sex hormones.

(b) Enzyme inhibition: A decrease in the drug metabolizing ability of an enzyme is called as enzyme inhibition. The process of inhibition may be direct or indirect.

Direct inhibition: It may result from interaction at the enzymic site bring out the change in enzyme activity. Direct enzyme inhibition can occur by one of the following mechanisms:

- **Competitive inhibition:** It occurs when structurally similar compounds compete for the same site on an enzyme. Example: Methacholine and acetylcholine compete for the enzyme cholinesterase which cause the inhibition of acetylcholine metabolism.
- **Non-competitive inhibition:** It occurs when a structurally unrelated agent interacts with the enzyme and prevents the metabolism of drugs. Example: Inhibition of phenytoin by isoniazid.
- **Product inhibition:** It occurs when the metabolic product competes with the substrate for the same enzyme.

Indirect inhibition: It is caused by one of the following mechanisms:

- **Repression:** It may be due to fall in the rate of enzyme synthesis or rise in the rate of enzyme degradation. Example: Due to the destruction of some enzyme by CCl_4, CS_2 etc.
- **Altered physiology:** It may be due to nutritional deficiency or hormonal imbalance.

(c) Environmental chemicals: Several environmental agents influence the drug metabolizing ability of enzymes.

Example: Halogenated pesticides such as DDT and polycyclic aromatic hydrocarbons contained in cigarette smoke have enzyme induction effect. Organophosphate insecticides and heavy metals such as mercury, nickel, cobalt and arsenic inhibit drug metabolizing ability of enzymes. Other environmental factors that may influence drug metabolism are temperature, altitude, pressure, atmosphere, etc.

Biological Factors:

(a) Age: The drug metabolic rate in the different age groups differs mainly due to variations in the enzyme content, enzyme activity and haemodynamics.

In neonates (upto 2 months) and in infants (2 months to 1 year), the microsomal enzyme system is not fully developed. So, many drugs are metabolized slowly. For example, caffeine has a half-life of 4 days in neonates in comparision to 4 hrs in adults.

Children (between 1 year and 12 years) metabolize several drugs much more rapidly than adults as the rate of metabolism reaches a maximum somewhere between 6 months and 12 years. As a result they require large mg/kg dose in comparison to adults.

In elderly persons, the liver size is reduced, the microsomal enzyme activity is decreased and hepatic blood flow also declines as a result of reduced cardiac output, all of which contributes to decreased metabolism of drugs. For example, chlomethiazole shows a high bioavailability within the elderly, therefore they require a lower dose.

(b) Diet: The enzyme content and activity is altered by a number of dietary components. Generally, low protein diet decreases and high protein diet increases the drug metabolizing ability as enzyme synthesis is promoted by protein diet and also raises the level of amino acids for conjugation with drugs.

Fat free diet depresses cytochrome P-450 levels since phospholipids, which are important components of microsomes become deficient.

Grapefruit inhibits metabolism of many drugs and improve their oral bioavailability.

Dietary deficiency of vitamins like Vitamin A, B2, B3, C and E) and minerals such as Fe, Ca, Mg, Zn retard the metabolic activity of enzymes.

Starvation results in decreased amount of glucuronides formed than under normal conditions.

(c) Sex difference: Since variations between male and female are observed following puberty. There is a related differences in the rate of metabolism may be due to sex hormones. Such sex differences were studied in rats which shows that male rats have greater drug metabolizing capacity than females. Example: In humans, women metabolize benzodiazepines slowly than men. Several studies have shown that women on contraceptive pills metabolize a number of drugs at a slow rate.

(d) Species difference: Species difference have been observed in both Phase-I and Phase-II reactions. In Phase-I reactions, both qualitative and quantitative variations in the enzyme and their activity have been observed. Qualitative differences among species generally result from the presence or absence of specific enzymes in those species. Quantitative differences result from variations in the amount and localization of enzymes, the amount of natural inhibitors, and the competition of enzymes for specific substrates.

Human liver contains less cytochrome P-450 per gram of tissue than do the livers of other species. For example, rat liver contains approximately 30 to 50 nmol/g of Cytochrome P450, whereas human liver contains 10 to 20 nmol/g. Furthermore, human liver is 2 percent of body weight, whereas rat liver is approximately 4 percent. Similarly, in men, amphetamine and ephedrine are predominantly metabolized by oxidative deamination, whereas in rats aromatic oxidation is the major route in Phase-II reactions. Similarly in pigs, the phenol is excreted mainly as glucuronide whereas its sulphate conjugate dominates in cats.

(e) Strain difference: The difference in drug metabolising ability between different species is related to genetics, the differences are observed between strains of same species also. It may be studied under two headings:

Pharmacogenetics: A study of inter-subject variability in drug response is called pharmacogenetics. The inter-subject variations in metabolism may either be monogenetically or polygenetically controlled. A polygenetic control is observed in twins. In identical twins (monozygotic), very little or no difference in metabolism of halothane, phenylbutazone, dicoumaral and antipyrine was detected but large variations were observed in fraternal twins (dizygotic).

Ethnic variations: Differences observed in the metabolism of drug among different races are called ethnic variations. Such variations may be monomorphic or polymorphic. **Example:** Approximately equal percent of slow and rapid acetylators are found among whites and blacks whereas the slow acetylators dominate Japanese and Eskimo population.

Physiological Factors:

- **Pregnancy:** Pregnancy is known to affect hepatic drug metabolism. Physiological changes during pregnancy are probably responsible for the reported alteration in drug metabolism. These 6 include elevated concentrations of various hormones such as estrogen, progesterone, placental growth hormones and prolactin. E.g. in women, the metabolism of promazine and pethidine is reduced during pregnancy.

- **Disease states:** There are many disease states that affect the metabolism of drugs. Some of them are cirrhosis of liver, alcoholic liver disease, cholestatic jaundice, diabetes mellitus, acromegaly, malaria, various bacterial and viral infections, etc. It can be seen that major effects are seen in the disease affecting liver as liver is quantitatively the important site for metabolism.

- **Hormonal imbalance:** Higher level of one hormone may inhibit the activity of few enzymes while inducing that of others. Example: Effect observed in the pituitary growth hormone and stress related changes in ACTH levels.

Physicochemical Properties of the Drug:

Molecular size and shape, pK_a, acidity/basicity, lipophilicity and steric and electronic characteristics of a drug influence in interaction with the active sites of enzyme and the metabolism to which it is subjected. However such an interrelationship is not clearly understood.

QUESTIONS

1. Discuss briefly solubility, partition coefficient, ionization and chelation in relation to biological action.
2. Add a note on protein binding.
3. Briefly discuss on various physicochemical parameters in relation to biological activity.
4. Discuss the role of bioisosterism in drug design.
5. Define the term drug metabolism. Enumerate various pathways for phase-I metabolism with suitable examples.
6. Discuss the importance of conjugation reaction in drug metabolism giving specific examples.
7. Explain phase-I and phase-II biotransformation.
8. Describe drug metabolism by oxidative and hydrolytic reactions giving example.
9. Discuss in brief the general pathway of drug metabolism.
10. Discuss the role of Cytochrome P-450 in drug metabolism.
11. Explain sites of drug biotransformation.

Unit ... *2*

DRUGS ACTING ON AUTONOMIC NERVOUS SYSTEM

♦ LEARNING OBJECTIVES ♦

After completing this unit, reader should be able to understand:

* ❖ To distinguish central nervous system from peripheral nervous system.
* ❖ To learn the autonomic nervous system in terms of its location and function.
* ❖ To learn the differences between the parasympathetic and sympathetic nervous systems.
* ❖ To learn biosynthesis, storage, release and metabolism of catecholamines.
* ❖ To learn various adrenergic receptors and their locations.
* ❖ To study various sympathomimetic drugs
* ❖ To study the synthesis of some selected adrenergic drugs.

2.1 INTRODUCTION

Adrenergic drug that mimic or interfere with the functioning of the sympathetic nervous system by affecting the release or action of norepinephrine and epinephrine. These hormones, which are also known as noradrenaline and adrenaline, are secreted by the adrenal gland, hence their association with the term *adrenergic*. The primary actions of norepinephrine and epinephrine are to mediate the "fight-or-flight response." Thus, they constrict blood vessels (vasoconstriction), which increases blood pressure, and accelerate the rate and force of contractions of the heart. Adrenergic drugs that produce or inhibit these effects are known as sympathomimetic agents and sympatholytic agents, respectively.

Therapeutically, these drugs are used to combat life-threatening disorders, which include acute attacks of bronchial asthma, shock, cardiac arrest, and allergic reactions. In addition these drugs are used as nasal decongestants and appetite suppressants.

2.2 ADRENERGIC NEUROTRANSMITTERS

The catecholamines are found in the body as norepinephrine, epinephrine, and dopamine are formed by hydroxylation and decarboxylation of the amino acids phenylalanine and tyrosine. All three of these catecholamines act as neurotransmitters in the central nervous system (CNS). Norepinephrine also functions as a neurotransmitter in the sympathetic nervous system. Although there are dopamine receptors outside the CNS, the role of dopamine as a hormone or neurotransmitter peripherally is not fully described. Epinephrine is the circulating hormone secreted by the adrenal medulla and influences processes throughout the body.

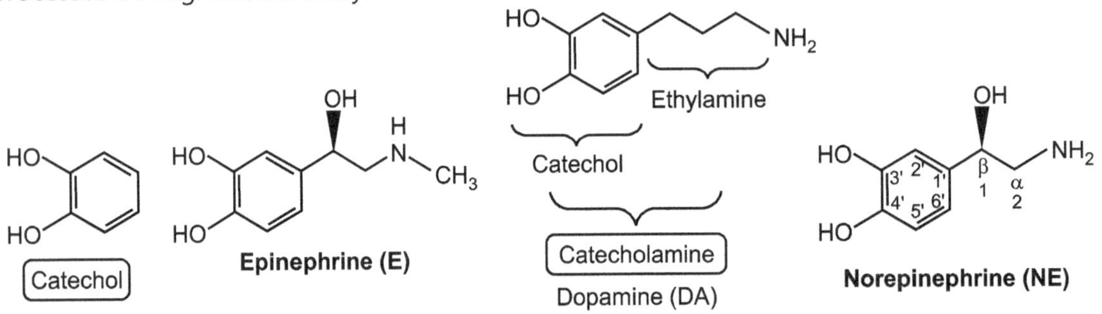

The catecholamines are 3, 4-dihydroxyphenolic amines. The benzene ring structure numbering is counter clockwise with carbon 1 being bonded to the aliphatic side chain. The catechol group consists of two adjacent hydroxyl groups: one at position 4, or para with respect to position 1 and the second at position 3, or ortho with respect to the hydroxyl at position 4. The aliphatic side-chain carbon atoms are labelled β and α. As illustrated, the substitutions on these carbons define each of the three most prominent catecholamines.

2.3 BIOSYNTHESIS AND CATABOLISM OF CATECHOLAMINES

2.3.1 Biosynthesis of Catecholamines

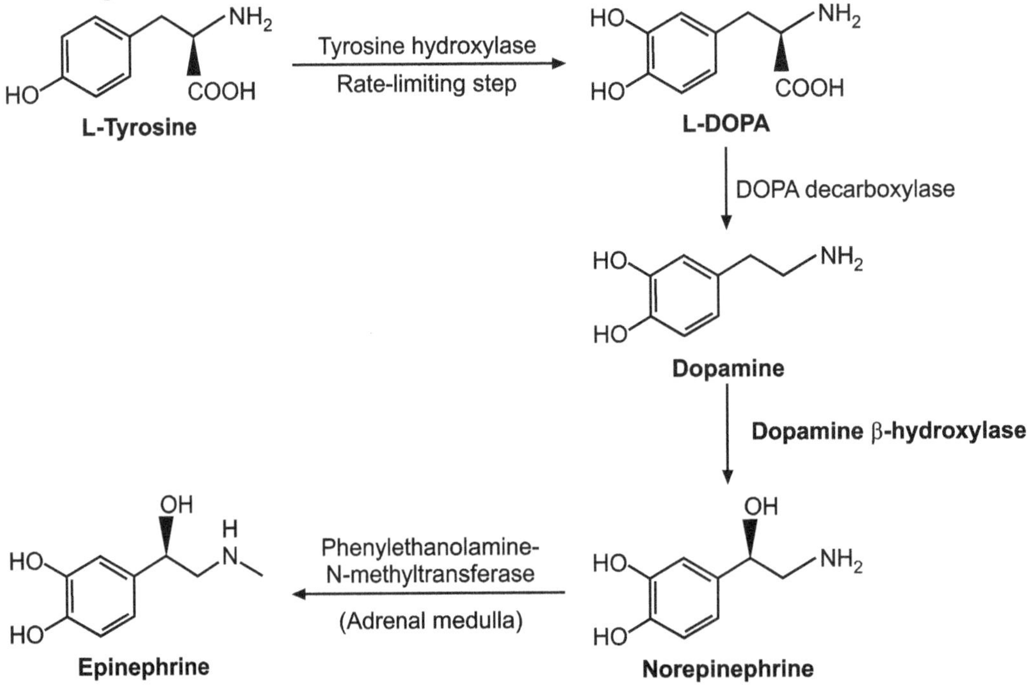

Biosynthesis begins with tyrosine, which consists of a benzene ring hydroxylated in the 4 (para) position to the two-carbon side chain at the 1 position. The β-carbon, closest to the ring, is saturated with hydrogen and is single bonded to the α-carbon. The α-carbon is bonded to the amino and carboxylic acid groups that define the amino acids. The rate-limiting enzyme, tyrosine hydroxylase, 3-hydroxylates (ortho with respect to the 4-position hydroxyl) tyrosine to dihydroxyphenylalanine (DOPA).

The α-carbon is decarboxylated by aromatic L-amino acid decarboxylase to form the first catecholamine, dopamine (L-dihydroxy phenylethylamine). Hydroxylation of the β-carbon of dopamine (by dopamine β-hydroxylase) results in the formation of norepinephrine. Dopamine β-hydroxylase requires vitamin C (ascorbic acid) as a cofactor.

Norepinephrine converted into epinephrine by methylation of the amino group on the α-carbon by phenylethanolamine-N-methyltransferase (PNMT). Tyrosine hydroxylase activity is the rate-limiting step in catecholamine synthesis.

The noradrenaline formed in the adrenergic nerve endings remain stored in vesicles as its adenosine triphosphate complex. The adrenal medulla also synthesizes and stores noradrenaline and adrenaline.

The neurotransmitters are released by increasing the permeability of nerve terminal membrane to Ca^{++}. The inflow of Ca^{++} triggers the fusion of vesicle with the cell membrane, resulting in exocytosis.

2.3.2 Catecholamine Catabolism

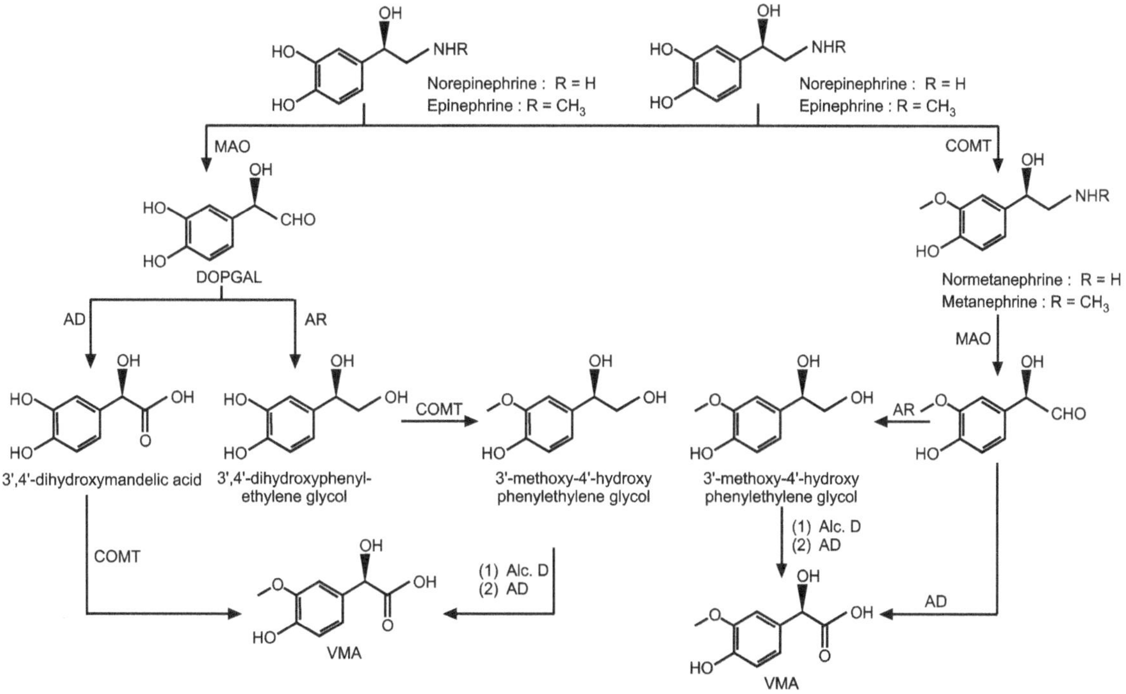

MAO = Monoamine oxidase, COMT = Catechol-O-methyltransferase, AD = Aldehyde dehydrogenase, Ak D = Alcohol dehydrogenase, DOPGAL = 3',4'-dihydrophenylglycoaldehyde, VMA = Vanillylmandelic acid, or 3-methoxy-4'-hydroxymandelic acid, AR = Aldehyde reluctase

There are two primary pathways for the degradation of catecholamines; one is near the site where catecholamines are synthesized and stored (chromaffin cells and sympathetic neurons), and the second deactivates primarily circulating catecholamines. Monoamine oxidase (MAO) catalyzes the first and catechol-O-methyltransferase (COMT). The second. MAO, a mitochrondrial enzyme, cleaves off the terminal aliphatic amine and oxidizes the α-carbon to carboxylic acid. The product, 3,4-dihydroxymandelic acid, is the same for epinephrine and norepinephrine because the N-methyl group that distinguishes the two is removed. COMT using the methyl-group donor S-adenosylmethionine methylates the 3-hydroxy group, producing metanephrine and normetanephrine, respectively, from epinephrine and norepinephrine. O-Methylation of 3,4-dihydroxymandelic acid by COMT or oxidative deamination of the metanephrines by MAO produces vanillylmandelic acid (VMA). Most of the substrates and products of these reactions may be conjugated to sulfate (primarily) or glucuronide, which reduces further metabolism and enhances excretion

2.4 ADRENERGIC RECEPTORS AND THEIR DISTRIBUTION

The two major categories of adrenergic receptors are designated alpha and beta which mediating the vasconstrictor actions of catecholamines. Alpha receptors have been further subdivided into:

- Receptor α_1 involves a Gq protein that elevates Ca^{++}, resulting in smooth muscle contraction. Receptor α_2 involves a Gi protein that decreases cAMP and C^{++} influx which inhibits neurotransmission.

- Receptors β_1, β_2 and β_3 involve a Gs protein and cAMP elevation that increases Ca^{++} for smooth muscle contraction (β_2 can be linked to a Gi protein that decreases cAMP resulting in smooth muscle relaxation). β_1 adrenoceptors occur in the heart and are involved in heart stimulation processes and its discharge. β_2 adrenoceptors appear in skeletal muscles and they stimulate the vasodilatations, Thus the effect of NE can be either excitatory or inhibitory, based on the receptor distribution within visceral organs.

2.5 SYMPATHOMIMETIC AGENTS (SM)

Sympathomimetic drug or adrenergic drugs are stimulant compounds which mimic the effects of endogenous catecholamines (adrenergic neurotransmitters) agonists of the sympathetic nervous system (i.e., epinephrine [adrenaline], norepinephrine [noradrenaline], and dopamine).

These agents include drugs that act on adrenergic receptors (adrenoceptors) directly or indirectly, such as by blocking the breakdown or neuronal uptake of catecholamines. Because sympathomimetic drugs raise blood pressure and increase heart rate, they are useful in treating systemic trauma, including bronchial asthma, shock, and cardiac arrest.

2.6 CLASSIFICATION OF SYMPATHOMIMETIC AGENTS

Sympathomimetic agents are classified as follows:

Direct acting: Nor-epinephrine, Epinephrine, Phenylepinephrine, Dopamine, Methyldopa, Clonidine, Dobutamine, Isoproterenol, Terbutaline, Salbutamol, Bitolterol, Naphazoline, Oxymetazoline and Xylometazoline.

Indirect acting: Hydroxyamphetamine, Psedoephedrine, Propylhexedrine.

Mixed acting: Ephedrine, Metaraminol.

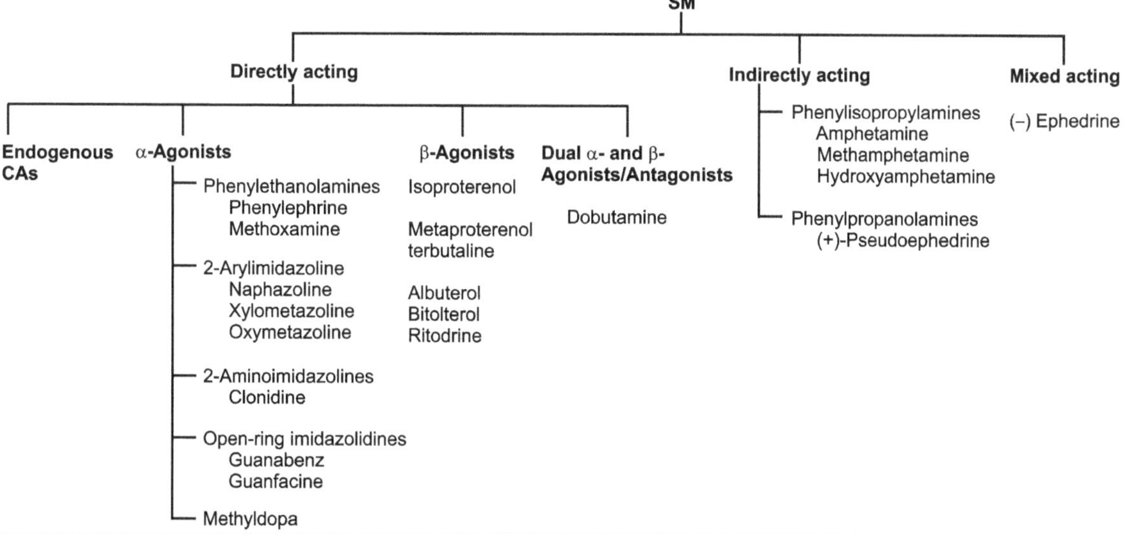

2.7 SAR OF SYMPATHOMIMETIC AGENTS

The parent structure of many adrenergic drugs is β-phenylethylamine.

- The modifications of β-phenylethylamine influence not only the mechanism of action, the receptor selectivity, but also their absorption, oral activity, metabolism, and thus duration of action (DOA).

- Naturally occurring catecholamine is active at both α and β-receptor but have a poor oral activity as it is rapidly metabolised by COMT. Thus the change in position of hydroxyl group from *meta* and *para* position to *meta* and *ortho* position gives a drug with good metabolic activity.

- For the direct-acting sympathomimetic amines, maximal activity is seen in β-phenylethylamine derivatives containing:

  o   catechol moiety and

  o   β-OH group on the ethylamine portion of the molecule.

- The greatest adrenergic activity occurs when two carbon atoms separate the aromatic ring from the amino group.

- For catecholamine, the more potent enantiomer has the (1R) configuration. This enantiomer is typically several 100 fold more potent than the enantiomer with the (1S) configuration.

- Primary and secondary amines have good adrenergic activity, whereas tertiary amines and quaternary ammonium salts do not.

- The nature of the amino substituent also affects the receptor selectivity of the compound. As the size of the nitrogen substituent increases, α-receptor agonist activity generally decreases and β-receptor agonist activity increases.

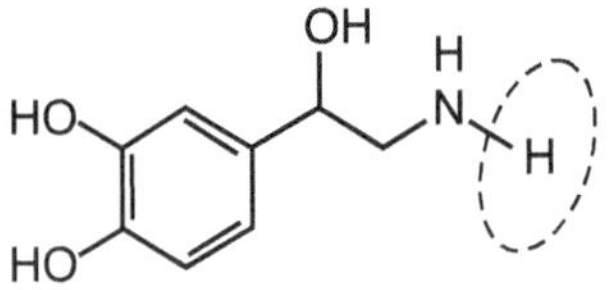

Norepinephrine (NE)
$\alpha > \beta$ **agonist**
α **agonist**

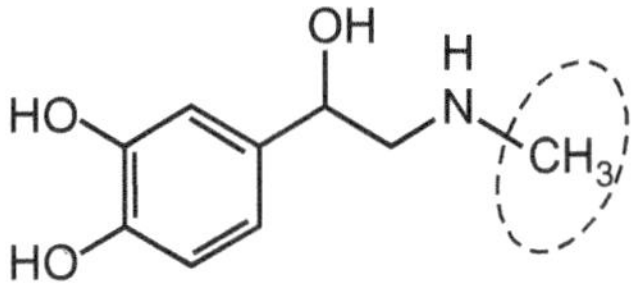

Epinephrine (E)
α, β_1 **and** β_2 **agonists**
non-selective α **and** β **agonists**

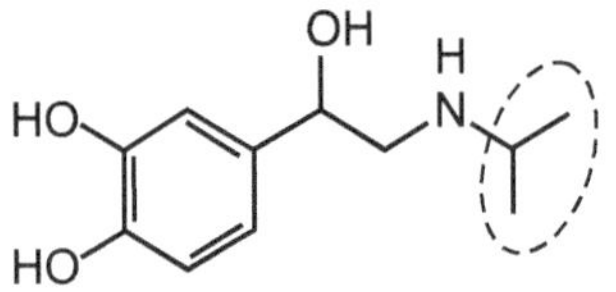

Isoproterenol (ISO)
β_1 **and** β_2 **agonists**
non-selective β **agonist**

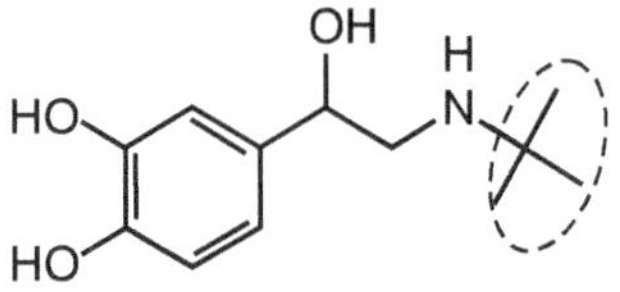

N-t-Butylnorepinephrine (Colterol)
selective β_2 **agonist**

- Thus, NE has more α-activity than β-activity and E is a potent agonist at α-, β_1-, and β_2-receptors. N-tert-butyl group enhances β_2-selectivity.

- Substitution on the α-carbon by small alkyl group (e.g., CH_3- or C_2H_5-) slows metabolism by MAO. This is very important for non-catechol compounds where the addition of small alkyl group increases the resistance to metabolism and lipophilicity, so such compounds often exhibit enhanced oral effectiveness and greater CNS activity than other compounds that do not contain an α-alkyl group.

- OH substitution on the β-carbon greatly enhances agonist activity at both α- and β-receptors and largely decreases CNS activity because it lowers lipid solubility.

- Maximal α- and β-activity depends on the presence of *meta* and *para* OH groups. Compounds without one or both phenolic OH substituents are not metabolized by COMT, and they are orally active and have longer duration of action. For example, phenylephrine (removal of *para* OH group, which lacks β action but has less α_1-agonist property).

Epinephrine

- Although the catechol moiety is important, maximal agonist activity at adrenoceptors, it can be replaced with other substituted phenyl moieties to provide selective adrenergic agonists. Replacement of the catechol moiety of isoprotenol with the resorcinol structure gives a selective β_2-agonist, which shows longer duration of action because they are resistant towards COMT.

Example: Metaproterenol

Metaproterenol

- Catecholamine without OH group on phenyl group (catechol moiety) loss of direct symathomimetic activity becomes indirectly sympathomimetic and not metabolised by COMT and they are orally active and have longer duration of action.

Example: Amphetamine.

Amphetamine

- A second chemical class of α-agonists is the imidazolines. These imidazolines are non-selective or can be selective for either α_1- or α_2-receptors. Structurally, most imidazolines have their heterocyclic imidazoline nucleus linked to a substituted aromatic moiety *via* some type of bridging unit. The optimum bridging unit (X) is usually a single methylene group or amino group.

Aromatic moiety { Ar — X — Imidazoline ring

Bridging unit

X = Usually CH_2 (α_1 agonists) or NH (α_2 agonists)

The optimum bridging unit (X) is usually a single methylene group or amino group.

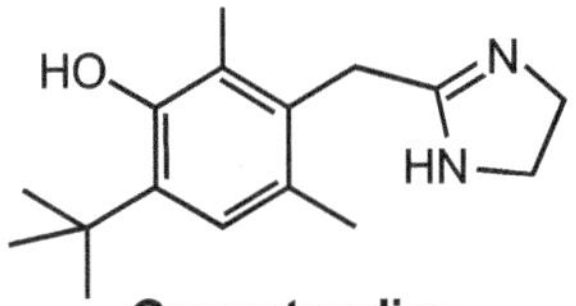

Oxymetazoline 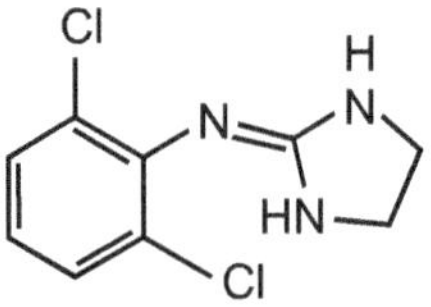   **Clonidine**

2.8 DIRECT ACTING SYMPATHOMIMETIC AGENTS

Direct acting drugs produce effect directly by interacting with adrenergic receptors and produce sympathomimetic effects. Structurally direct acting adrenergic agonist contain catechol moiety (i.e. OH group at both *meta* and *para* position) along with OH group at β-position and lacks of α-position substitution in side chain. These compounds are easily metabolised by both MAO and COMT.

Direct-acting sympathomimetics are classified based on their selectivity for adrenoceptors, of which there are several types, including α_1, α_2, β_1 and β_2 substances that activate β_2-adrenoceptors (known as β_2-adrenoceptor agonists) are some of the most widely used direct-acting sympathomimetics, especially in the treatment of asthma because of their ability to relax smooth muscle tissue in the airways of the lungs. However, none of the available drugs are completely selective for the β_2-adrenoceptor, and they tend to produce unwanted effects on the heart, such as increased heart rate and disturbances of cardiac rhythm, through their action on cardiac β_1-adrenoceptors. To reduce these side effects, the β_2 agonists are usually given by inhalation, which increases pulmonary exposure to the drug while lowering systemic exposure and therefore activation of cardiac receptors. Examples of β_2 agonists include terbutaline, albuterol, and metaproterenol. Some direct-acting agents are nonselective; for example, isoproterenol produces effects at all β receptors, and the (+) and (−) isoforms of dobutamine produce varying effects at α and β receptors.

2.8.1 Epinephrine (Adrenaline)

Epinephrine is a naturally occurring cathecholamine, direct-acting sympathomimetic agent exerting its effect on alpha and beta adrenoreceptors. It is a powerful cardiac stimulant.

- α stimulation causes peripheral, renal, splanchnic and pulmonary vasoconstriction.
- β_1 stimulation causes an increase in heart rate, contractility and excitability.
- β_2 stimulation causes an increase in bronchodilation and vasodilation in skeletal muscles.
- It is administered in cardiac arrest to cause peripheral vasoconstriction via its alphaadrenergic action (increases available cardiac output to myocardium and brain).
- It may facilitate defibrillation by improving myocardial blood flow during CPR.

Epinephrine is chemically, (R)1-(3,4-dihydroxyphenyl)-2-methylaminoethanol. (R)-epinephrine is 12 times more potent than (S)-form. Major effects are increased systolic blood pressure, reduced diastolic pressure, tachycardia, hyperglycaemia and hypokalaemia. It has vasopressor properties, an antihistaminic action and is a bronchodilator.

Epinephrine (Adrenaline)

Adrenaline is rapidly distributed to the heart, spleen, several glandular tissues and adrenergic nerves. It crosses the placenta and is excreted in breast milk. It is approximately 50% bound to plasma proteins. The onset of action is rapid and after intravenous infusion the half life is approximately 5-10 minutes. Adrenaline is rapidly metabolised in the liver and tissues. Upto 90% of the IV dose is excreted as metabolites in the urine due to rapid oxidation and conjugation by both COMT and MAO.

Uses:

It is used as sympathomimetics, broncholytis and antiasthamatics. It prevents internal bleeding during surgery. Used to treat heart blocks and open angle glaucoma. Also used in emergencies to treat serious allergic reactions to insect stings/bites, foods, drugs, or other substances. It improves breathing, stimulates the heart, raises a dropping blood pressure, reduce swelling of the face, lips, and throat.

Adverse Effects:

Tachycardia, anxiety, restlessness, tremor, weakness, dizziness, headache, nausea, vomiting, flushing and redness of face and skin, hypertension and increased after load, exacerbation of myocardial ischaemia, renal vasoconstriction may reduce renal blood flow and glomerular filtration rate, hypokalaemia and hyperglycaemia.

2.8.2 Nor-epinephrine (Nor-adrenaline)

Nor-epinephrine is a natural catecholamine and a phenethylamine derivative. It differs from adrenaline only by lacking the methyl substitution on the aminoethanol and, as for adrenaline. Chemically it is 1-β-[3,4-dihydroxyphenyl]-α-aminoethanol. The L-isomer is pharmacologically active and potent α_1- receptor agonist but has a relatively less β_2-receptor activity. It functions as a peripheral vasoconstrictor (alpha-adrenergic action) and as an inotropic stimulator of the heart and dilator of coronary arteries (beta-adrenergic action). Along with epinephrine, norepinephrine also underlies the fight-or-flight response, directly increasing heart rate, triggering the release of glucose from energy stores, and increasing blood flow to skeletal muscle.

Norepinephrine is synthesized from dopamine by dopamine β-hydroxylase. It is released from the adrenal medulla into the blood as a hormone, and is also a neurotransmitter in the central nervous system and sympathetic nervous system where it is released from noradrenergic neurons. The actions of norepinephrine are carried out via the binding to adrenergic receptors.

Noradrenaline is predominantly metabolised by catechol-o-methyltransferase (COMT) and monoamine oxidase (MAO). Noradrenaline has a rapid onset of action (1-2 minutes), and a fast elimination when the infusion is ceased due to the short half-life of 1-2 minutes.

Norepinephrine (Noradrenaline)

Mechanism of Action:

Norepinephrine is synthesized from tyrosine as a precursor, and packed into synaptic vesicles. It performs its action by being released into the synaptic cleft, where it acts on adrenergic receptors, followed by the signal termination, either by degradation of norepinephrine, or by uptake by surrounding cells.

Biosynthesis:

Norepinephrine is synthesized by a series of enzymatic steps in the adrenal medulla and postganglionic neurons of the sympathetic nervous system from the amino acid tyrosine.

- The first reaction is the hydroxylation into dihydroxyphenylalanine (L-DOPA) (DOPA = 3,4-DiHydroxy-L-Phenylalanine), catalyzed by tyrosine hydroxylase. This is the rate-limiting step.

- This is followed by decarboxylation into the neurotransmitter dopamine, catalyzed by pyridoxal phosphate and DOPA decarboxylase.

- Last is the final β-oxidation into norepinephrine by dopamine beta hydroxylase, requiring ascorbate as a cofactor (electron donor).

Uses:

Norepinephrine is similar to adrenaline used for blood pressure control in certain acute hypotensive states (e.g., pheochromocytomectomy, sympathectomy, poliomyelitis, spinal anesthesia, myocardial infarction, septicemia, blood transfusion, and drug reactions).

Adverse Effects:

Ischaemic injury due to potent vasoconstrictor action and tissue hypoxia, bradycardia, anxiety, transient headache, respiratory difficulty.

2.8.3 Phenylepinephrine

Phenylephrine hydrochloride is a synthetic sympathomimetic agent. Chemically, phenylephrine hydrochloride is (-)-m-Hydroxy-α-[(methylamino)methyl]benzyl alcohol. It differs from adrenaline only by the absence of hydroxyl group on *para* position on the aromatic ring.

- It is potent vasoconstriction and is active when given orally because it is resistant to COMT and active orally.
- It is a selective direct acting α_1-receptor agonist.
- Its duration of action is about twice that of epinephrine.
- Due to lack of catechol moiety, it is not metabolised by COMT, but metabolised by MAO.
- Relatively non-toxic and produce little CNS stimulation.

1-(3-hydroxyphenyl)-2-methylamino ethanol

Synthesis: Synthesised by treating phenol with chloroacetyl chloride under acidic conditions. Later treated with methyl amine and then reduced and resolved with sulphonate derivative to yield phenylepinephrine.

Phenol + **Chloroacetyl chloride** $\xrightarrow{-HCl}$ **m-hydroxy phenyl acetyl chloride**

$\xrightarrow{CH_3NH_2}$

(i) H_2/catalytic reduction
(ii) Resolved with α-camphor sulphonate

(–) Phenylephrine

Uses: It reduces congestion and swelling by constricting the blood vessels of the membrane. It dilates the pupil and used to treat open angle glaucoma.

2.8.4 Dopamine

Chemically it is 2-(3,4-dihydroxy phenyl)-1-amino ethane. It is ineffective orally as it acts as a substrate for both MAO and COMT. It acts on β_2-adrenergic receptor and cause positive ionotropic effects and also causes the release of nor-epinephrine.

Dopamine

Uses:

It increases blood flow to the kidneys. It exerts CVS effect by interacting with D_1-dopaminergic receptors especially in the mesenteric, renal and coronary beds. Also in heart attack, trauma, surgery and other serious medical conditions.

2.8.5 Methyldopa

Chemically it is (2S)-2-amino-3-(3,4-dihydroxyphenyl)-2-methylpropanoic acid. It is used as a prodrug, it is metabolised by enzymes and gives active metabolite α-methyl norepinephrine which is α_2 agonist acting in the CNS thereby decreases the sympathetic outflow leads to lower blood pressure. It is a drug of choice for treating hypertension during pregnancy.

Methyldopate → (Esterase) → **L-α-Methyldopa** → (DOPA decarboxylase) → **α-Methyldopamine** → (Dopamine β-hydroxylase) → **(1R,2S)-α-Methylnorepinephrine selective α_2-agonist**

Uses:

This medication is used alone or with other medications to treat high blood pressure (hypertension). Lowering high blood pressure helps prevent strokes, heart attacks, and kidney problems. Methyldopa works by relaxing blood vessels so blood can flow more easily.

2.8.6 Clonidine

Clonidine is an example of 2-aminoimidazoline derivatives. Chemically, it is N-(2,6-dichlorophenyl)-4,5-dihydro-1H-imidazol-2-amine that possess selective α_2-adrenergic receptor. Inductive and resonance effect of dichlorophenyl ring decreases the pK_a of clonidine. Clonidine enters the CNS and stimulate α_2-receptor located in the brain. Thus decreases the peripherial vascular resistance (PVR) and decreases the blood pressure and heart rate.

It inhibits both dopaminergic and adrenergic neurotransmitter by inhibiting DOPA decarboxylase which converts L-Dopa into dopamine. Clonidine should normally be used in those patients in whom treatment with diuretic or beta-blocker was found ineffective

Clonidine (pK_a = 8.0)

Mechanism of Action:

Clonidine hydrochloride is an α adrenergic agonist which also has some α adrenergic antagonist effects. The antihypertensive effect of clonidine hydrochloride is thought to be due to central α_2 adrenergic stimulation, which results in a decreased sympathetic outflow to the heart, kidneys, and peripheral vasculature and thus decreased peripheral vascular resistance, decreased systolic and diastolic blood pressure and decreased heart rate.

Uses:

Treatment of hypertension, nasal decongestant, open eye glaucoma. It is a potent sedative-hypnotic drug and can prevent post-operative shivering.

2.8.7 Dobutamine

Dobutamine is a synthetic catecholamine and act as dual α and β-agonists/antagonists that stimulate beta receptors of the heart to produce mild chronotropic, hypertensive, arrhythmogenic and vasodilative effects. Chemically it is an analogue of dopamine in which, 1-methyl-3-(4-hydroxyphenyl)propyl substituent has been replaced on the amino group.

It possesses an asymmetric carbon atom and exhibits as a pair of enantiomers.

- The (+) enantiomer possessing a potent full agonist activity at both β_1 and β_2-receptors but (+) isomer is a potent α_1 antagonist.

- The (−) enantiomer posseses a potent agonist activity at α_1-receptors and 10 times less potent at β_1 and β_2-receptors.

- It can be metabolised by COMT and conjugation but not by MAO.

Dobutamine

It stimulates the beta receptors in the heart and produces mild chronotropic, hypertensive, arrhythmogenic and vasodilative effects. It stimulates the beta -1 stimulation results in an increase in heart rate (mild), myocardial contractility and excitability. Beta-2 stimulation is minimal and may have some peripheral vasodilatation and brochodilation. The onset of action is within 1-2 minutes, but with an infusion it may take upto 10 minutes to obtain the peak effect.

Uses:

It is used in the ICU for the treatment of congestive heart failure, cardiogenic shock, pulmonary oedema and to increase cardiac output. It is less arrythmogenic than adrenaline.

2.8.8 Isoproterenol (Isoprenaline)

Isoproterenol hydrochloride is 3,4-Dihydroxy-α-[(isopropylamino)methyl] benzyl alcohol hydrochloride, a synthetic sympathomimetic amine that is structurally related to epinephrine but acts almost exclusively on beta receptors. Isoproterenol hydrochloride is a racemic compound. It is a potent non-selective and a synthetic catecholamine with β-adrenergic receptor agonist and with very low affinity for alpha-adrenergic receptors.

Isoproterenol (Isoprenaline)

It acts on both β_1 and β_2 receptor and does not act on α-receptors. It increases the cardiac output by stimulating β-receptor and bronchodilation by stimulating β_2-receptor located on the respiratory tract. It is available as inhalator, injections and sublingual tablets. It is not taken orally due to less or no oxidation deamination by MAO. It undergoes metabolism by COMT. It is synthesised by following method.

4-Chloroacetylcatechol   **Isopropylamine**

Isoproterenol

Uses:

It is used in the treatment of bronchial asthma, an antiarrhythmic agent, CNS stimulant and peripherial vasodilator. Also used in the treatment of shock to increase the heart rate.

Adverse Effects:

CNS: Nervousness, headache, dizziness, nausea, visual blurring.

Cardiovascular: Tachycardia, palpitations, angina, Adams-Stokes attacks, pulmonary edema, hypertension, hypotension, ventricular arrhythmias, tachyarrhythmias.

Respiratory: Dyspnea.

2.8.9 Terbutaline

Terbutaline is a non-catecholamine, therefore is resistant to COMT. Chemically terbutaline is N-tert-butyl-N-[2-(3,5-dihydroxyphenyl)-2-hydroxymethyl] amine. It is a selective β_2-adrenergic receptor agonist resulting in smooth muscle relaxation. It is a fast acting bronchodilator.

Terbutaline is prepared by reduction of 2-(tert-butylamino)-3', 5'-dihydroxyacetophenone by catalytic hydrogenation.

Terbutaline

The effect of this medicine can be observed within 30-45 minutes and effective for upto 4-8 hours upon oral administration.

Uses:

Terbutaline is a bronchodilator medicine that is used to relieve symptoms such as wheezing, shortness of breath, chest tightness, breathing difficulties, coughing etc. associated with asthma. It is used to treat an acute attack of asthma as well as for prevention of further asthma attacks.

2.8.10 Salbutamol (Albuterol)

Salbutamol or albuterol are selective beta-2-adrenergic bronchodilator and structurally is replacement of the *meta* OH of the catechol structure with a hydroxymethyl group. Salbutamol is sold as a racemic mixture. The (R)-(−)-enantiomer is responsible for the pharmacologic activity; the (S)-(+)-enantiomer blocks metabolic pathways. Chemically, it is (RS)-4-[2-(tert-butylamino)-1-hydroxyethyl]-2-(hydroxymethyl) phenol. It is resistant towards MAO and COMT metabolism due to the presence of hydroxymethyl moiety and bulky N-substitutions.

Salbutamol (Albuterol)

Salbutamol is a bronchodilator, β_2 adrenoreceptor stimulant, with some β_1 effects at high dosage levels.

- β_1 stimulation causes an increase in heart rate, contractility and excitability.
- β_2 stimulation causes bronchodilatation and vasodilatation.
- It causes uterine smooth muscle relaxation and is used to help prevent premature labour.

Mechanism of Action:

The prime action of beta-adrenergic drugs is to stimulate adenyl cyclase, the enzyme which catalyzes the formation of cyclic-3',5'-adenosine monophosphate (cyclic AMP) from adenosine triphosphate (ATP). The cyclic AMP thus formed mediates the cellular responses.

Salbutamol is prepared from an acetophenone derivative as follows:

Uses:

This drug relaxes the smooth muscle in the lungs and opens airways to improve breathing. It is used to treat asthma, chronic bronchitis and emphysema.

2.8.11 Bitolterol

Bitolterol, (3-4 diester colterol) is a new β_2-adrenergic agonist. Since it is itself biologically inactive, bitolterol is considered a pro-drug. When administered it is activated within the lung by esterase hydrolysis to the active compound colterol catecholamine N-t-butyl-arterenol). Chemically, it is [4-(1-Hydroxy-2-tert-butylamino-ethyl)-2-(4-methylbenzoyl)oxy-phenyl] 4-methylbenzoate. The presence of two p-toluic acids made the drug more lipophilic than the parent drug. It has a longer duration of action than isoproterenol and metabolised by COMT and conjugation.

Bitolterol (a prodrug of colterol)

Esterases in the lung and other tissues

Colterol　　　　**p-Toluic acid**

Mechanism of Action:

Bitolterol is an adrenergic beta-2 agonist. Asthma results from a narrowing of the bronchial tubes. This narrowing is caused by muscle spasm and inflammation within the bronchial tubes. Agonist of the beta-2 adrenergic receptors by bitolterol leads to relaxation of smooth muscles surrounding these airway tubes which then increase the diameter and ease of air flow through the tubes.

Uses:

In bronchial asthma and reversible bronchospasm.

2.8.12 Naphazoline

Naphazoline is a rapid and direct acting sympathomimetic drug and exists in an ionised form at physiological pH due to the basic nature of imidazole ring (pH = 9-10). Chemically it is 2-(1-naphthylmethyl)-2-imidazoline and an imidazoline derivative. It is partial agonist at both α_1 and α_2-adrenergic receptors. Lipophilic substituents on the phenyl ring are important for α_1-selectivty. Naphazoline is used to induce systemic vasoconstriction, thereby decreasing nasal congestion and inducing constriction around the conjunctiva and also constricts the smaller arterioles of nasal passages, producing a decongesting effect. Naphazoline ophthalmic causes constriction of blood vessels in eyes. It also decreases itching and irritation of eyes. It is prepared by strong heating of 1-naphthaleneacetonitrile with ethylenediamine monochloride at 200°C.

Naphazoline

Uses:

It is used as a local vasoconstrictor for the relief of nasal congestion due to allergic manifestation. Used for the relief of ocular congestion and blepharospasm.

2.8.13 Oxymetazoline

Oxymetazoline is direct acting sympathomimetic drug. Chemically it is 3-(4,5-dihydro-1H-imidazol-2-ylmethyl)-2,4-dimethyl-6-tert-butyl-phenol and shows selective α_2-receptor agonist activity.

Ethylene diamine

Acetonitrile   **Oxylometazoline**

Uses: As a topical decongestant in the form of nasal spray (Otrivin).

2.8.14 Xylometazoline

Chemically, it is 2-[(4-tert-butyl-2,6-dimethylphenyl)methyl]-4,5-dihydro-1H-imidazole. It is selective α_2-adrenergic receptor and stimulates the blood vessels of nose.

Xylometazoline

Uses:

As a decongestant during the allergy or infection of the nasal passage.

2.9 INDIRECT ACTING SYMPATHOMIMETIC AGENTS

Indirect-acting sympathomimetic drugs are those that act indirectly to increase the concentration of the endogenous neurotransmitter by causing release of endogenous NE. These drugs enter the nerve ending by active uptake and displace NE from its storage granules.

This class is of non-catecholamines, they are similar to phenylethylamine with some structural modifications. These compounds are resistant to COMT and MAO enzymes due to lack of phenolic hydroxyl groups and presence of α-methyl groups. These compounds pass more readily through blood brain barrier because of increased lipophilicity.

2.9.1 Hydroxyamphetamine

Hydroxyamphetamine are indirect sympathomimetic agents and derivative of amphetamines i.e. a metabolic product of amphetamine. It is chemically 4-(2-aminopropyl) phenol. It is an α-receptor and stimulates the sympathetic nervous system.

Hydroxyamphetamine

Mechanism of Action:

Hydroxyamphetamine hydrobromide is an indirect acting sympathomimetic agent which causes the release of norepinephrine from adrenergic nerve terminals.

4-hydroxyamphetamine

4-hydroxynorephedrine

Amphetamine

Norephedrine

4-hydroxyphenylacetone   Phenylacetone   Benzoic acid   Hippuric acid

Metabolic Pathways of Amphetamine in Humans:

Uses:

It is a sympathomimetic and anticholinergic combination and relaxes muscles of the eye by dilating the pupil (mydriasis). In narcolepsy (sudden attack of sleep in completely inappropriate situations). Also used in children with hyperkinetic syndrome and in the treatment of obesity.

2.9.2 Psedoephedrine

Chemically. it is (S,S)-2-methylamino-1-phenylpropan-1-ol. Pseudoephedrine is a diasteromer of ephedrine and get oxidised to methcathinone or reduced into methamphetamine. Whereas ephedrine has a mixed mechanism of action, L-(+)- pseudoephedrine and acts mostly by an indirect mechanism and has virtually no direct activity. The structural basis for this difference in mechanism is the stereochemistry of the carbon atom possessing the β-OH group. It is sympathomimetic agent and put direct effect on adrenergic receptors. (α-adrenergic receptors present on the walls of blood vessel).

Pseudoephedrine

Uses:

Used as vasoconstrictor, to treat nasal and sinus congestion, or congestion of the tubes that drain fluid from your inner ears.

2.9.3 Propylhexedrine

Chemically it is (±)-1-cyclohexyl-N-methylpropan-2-amine. It is an analogue of amphetamine in which the aromatic ring has been replaced by the cyclohexane ring. It produces vasoconstriction and decongestant effect. It inhibits MAO and metabolised by COMT and thus increases NE to show the sympathetic activity.

Methamphetamine   **Propylhexedrine**

Uses:

It is used for the relief of congestion due to colds, allergies and allergic rhinitis and its euphoric effects.

2.10 MIXED ACTING SYMPATHOMIMETIC AGENTS

Mixed-acting adrenergic agonists are compounds that cause activation of adrenergic receptors by both direct binding as well as release of endogenously-stored norepinephrine from presynaptic terminals. Ephedrine is the prototype mixed-acting agonist. They have no hydroxyls on the aromatic ring but do have a β-hydroxyl group.

2.10.1 Ephedrine

Chemically, it is 2-methylamino-1-phenyl propan-1-ol. It has both α and β-adrenergic agonistic effect. Ephedrine is a central nervous system stimulant. It is not metabolized by either MAO or COMT and therefore has more oral activity and longer duration of action than E. Ephedrine has two asymmetric carbon atoms, so it has four isomers. D(-) isomer is the most active of the four isomers as a presser amine because it has the correct (1R,2S) configuration for optimal direct action at adrenergic receptors. Lacking phenolic OH groups, ephedrine is less polar and thus crosses the BBB far better than do other CAs.

Enantiomers

Ephedrine
(threo cacemate)
Mix acting drug

(−) Ephedrine   **(+) Ephedrine**

Uses:

Used as bronchodilator, nasal decongestant, orthostatic hypotension or myasthenia gravis.

2.10.2 Metaraminol

Chemically, it is 3-[-2-amino-1-hydroxy-propyl] phenol. It is an α-adrenergic receptor agonist with some β-receptor effect. It has mixed mechanism of action and can be used parenterally as vasopressor in prevention of acute hypertension state occurring with spinal anaesthesia.

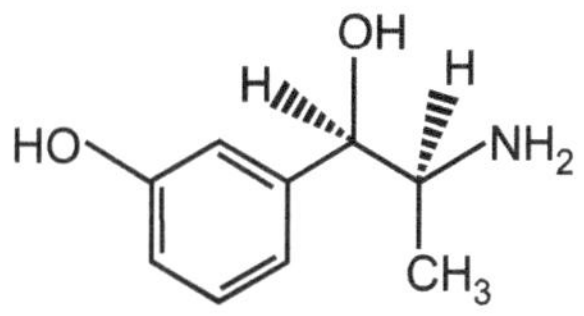

Metaraminol

Uses:

It is a potent sympathomimetic amine used in the prevention and treatment of hypotension, particularly as a complication of anaesthesia.

2.11 ADRENERGIC ANTAGONISTS / ADRENEROLYTIC

A sympatholytic (or adrenerolytic) drug is a medication which inhibits transmission of impulses from the postganglionic functioning of the sympathetic nervous system or inhibiting the transmission of nerve impulses in the sympathetic nervous system.

They can block at three different levels:

- Peripheral sympatholytic drugs (α and β receptor antagonists) block the action of NA at the effector organ (heart or blood vessel).

- Ganglionic blockers that block impulse transmission at the sympathetic ganglia.

- Centrally acting sympatholytic drugs that block sympathetic activity within the brain.

2.12 CLASSIFICATION OF ADRENEROLYTIC / SYMPATHOLYTIC (SL)

SL

α-Antagonists

β-Antagonists

Non-selective

Selective α_1-Antagonists

Selective α_2-Antagonists

Reversible
- Imidazolines
  Tolazoline
  Phentolamine

Irreversible
- β-Haloalkylamines
  Dibenamine
  Phenoxybenzamin

- Quinazolines
  Prazosin
  Terazosin
  Doxazosin
  Alfuzosin
- Tamsulosin

- Indole alkylamine alkaloid
  Yohimbine

Non-selective (First generation)
- Propranolol

Selective β_1-Antagonists (Second generation) (Cardioselective β-blockers)
- Atenolol
- Betaxolol
- Bisoprolol
- Esmolol

Mixed α/β-Antagonists (Third generation)
- Labetalol
- Carvedilol

2.13 ALPHA (α)-ADRENERGIC ANTAGONISTS / (α)-ADRENERGIC BLOCKERS

Adrenergic blocker agents prevent the response of effector organs to endogenous as well as exogenous adrenaline and nor-adrenaline.

Alpha receptor is one of the two receptors through which the sympathetic nervous system. The α-adrenergic receptors are further subdivided into two distinct types: α_1, most of which are located post-junctionally on the vascular smooth muscle cell producing vasoconstriction and α_2, which are located prejunctionally on the sympathetic nerve ending having negative feedback on norepinephrine release into the synapse.

2.13.1 Tolazoline

Tolazoline belongs to the synthetic non-selective competitive alpha-adrenergic blocking agents known as imidazoline derivative. It is a mixed alpha-1 and alpha-2 adrenergic receptor antagonist. Chemically it is 1H-Imidazole, 4,5-dihydro-2-(phenylmethyl) mono-hydrochloride and structurally similar to the imidazoline α-agonist like nephazole and xylometazoline.

Synthesis:

It is prepared by condensation of an amino ether (obtained by methanolysis of phenylacetonitrile) with ethylene diamine.

$$C_6H_5-CH_2-CN \longrightarrow \text{(phenyl)}-CH_2-C\underset{NH}{\overset{OCH_3}{|}} \quad \xrightarrow{H_2N-CH_2-CH_2-NH_2} \quad \text{Tolazoline}$$

Use:

Tolazoline has been used in the treatment of persistant pulmonary hypertension of the newborn.

2.13.2 Phentolamine

Phentolamine is a reversible non-selective α-adrenergic antagonist. Chemically it is 3-[(4,5-Dihydro-1H-imidazol-2-ylmethyl)(4-methylphenyl)amino]phenol. It is an imidazoline derivative and causes vasodilation and alters the effect of adrenergic drug.

Synthesis:

N-(4-methylphenyl)-3-hydroxyaniline on condensation with hydrogen cyanide and formaldehyde gives N-(4-methylphenyl)-3-hydroxy anilinoacetonitrile which on further treatment with ethylene diamine gives phentolamine.

Uses: It is used in the treatment of hypertension and hypertensive emergencies, pheochromocytoma, vasospasm of Raynaud disease. As a drug of choice when no responds to benzodiazepines and calcium-channel blockers.

2.13.3 Phenoxybenzamine

Phenoxybenzamine is a non-selective, irreversible alpha blocker having long duration of action because it forms a permanent covalent bond with adrenergic receptors. It has been used to treat hypertension and as a peripheral vasodilator. Chemically, it is benzyl-N-(2-chloroethyl)-1-phenoxypropan-2-amine. It also blocks acetylcholine, histamine and serotonine receptor and shows vasodilatory effect.

Phenoxybenzamine

Drugs   **Aziridinium ion**   **Alkylated receptor**

Uses:

Used to treat hypertension caused by pheochromocytoma and pulmonary oedema.

2.13.4 Prazosin

Chemically, it is [4-(4-Amino-6,7-dimethoxy-2-quinazolinyl)-1-piperazinyl](2-furyl) methanone. It is quninazoline derivative, piperazine ring with acyl moiety. It is a highly selective competitive antagonist of the α_1-adrenergic receptor. It lowers the blood pressure, heart rate and cardiac output.

Effects of Prazosin and Analogs on the Cardiovascular System:

* Prazosin and its analogs are selective α_1-receptor blockers used to treat hypertension. These agents have similar cardiovascular actions, differing only in pharmacokinetic parameters. Doxazosin, trimazosin and terazosin are more widely used than prazosin.

- These agents relax the smooth muscle associated with arteries and veins.

- This results in decrease in systemic arterial blood pressure due to decrease in peripheral vascular resistance and venous return.

- The reduction in arterial blood pressure **does not** result in a significant increase in heart rate.

- Treatment with these drugs can result in fluid retention as a response to the lowering of blood pressure. Thus the drugs can be prescribed with a diuretic in the treatment of hypertension.

- May have beneficial effects on lipid profiles by increasing HDL cholesterol and decreasing LDL cholesterol.

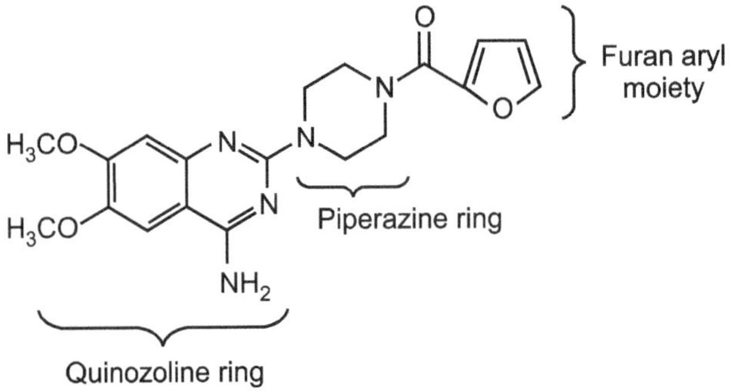

Uses: Hypertension, Raynaud's disease.

2.13.5 Dihydroergotamine

It is an ergot alkaloid and is a derivative of lysergic acid. It is a semi-synthetic form of ergotamine. It affects adrenoreceptors, DA and 5-histamine receptors. It possesses α-agonistic and vasoconstrictor actions.

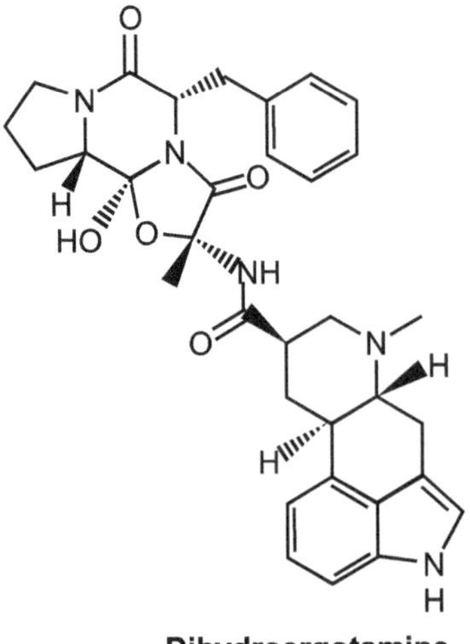

Dihydroergotamine

Mechanism of Action:

Dihydroergotamine binds with high affinity to $5\text{-HT}_{1D\alpha}$ and $5\text{-HT}_{1D\beta}$ receptors. It also binds with high affinity to serotonin 5-HT_{1A}, 5-HT_{2A}, and 5-HT_{2C} receptors, noradrenaline α_{2A}, α_{2B} and α, receptors, and dopamine D_{2L} and D_3 receptors.

The therapeutic activity of dihydroergotamine in migraine is generally attributed to the agonist effect at 5-HT_{1D} receptors. Two current theories have been proposed to explain the efficacy of 5-HT_{1D} receptor agonists in migraine. One theory suggests that activation of 5-HT_{1D} receptors located on intracranial blood vessels leads to vasoconstriction, which correlates with the relief of migraine headache. The alternative hypothesis suggests that activation of 5-HT_{1D} receptors on sensory nerve endings of the trigeminal system results in the inhibition of pro-inflammatory neuropeptide release.

Uses: Effective in headache and severe migraine pain. It can be administered by IV, subcutaneously or by nasal spray.

2.13.6 Methysergide

Methysergide is a partially synthetic compound structurally related to lysergic acid butanolamide, well known as methylergonovine. Chemically, methysergide maleate is designated as ergoline-8-carboxamide, 9,10-didehydro-N-[1-(hydroxymethyl)propyl]-1,6-dimethyl-(8b)-(Z)-2-butenedioate. Methylation in the number 1 position of the ring structure enormously enhances the antagonism to serotonin that is present to a much lesser degree in the partially methylated compound (methylergonovine maleate) as well as altering other pharmacologic properties.

Methysergide

Mechanism of Action:

Methysergide is serotonin antagonist and acts on central nervous system (CNS), which directly stimulates the smooth muscle leading to vasoconstriction. Some alpha-adrenergic blocking activity has been reported. Suggestions have been made by investigators as to the mechanism whereby methysergide produces its clinical effects, but this has not been finally established, although it may be related to the antiserotonin effect.

Uses:

To treat chronic migraine and cluster headache (prevention or reduction) of intensity and frequency of vascular headaches

2.14 BETA (β)-ADRENERGIC BLOCKERS

These agents antagonise the effect of the catecholamine at α and β-adrenergic receptor. They block the effects of endogenous and exogenous catecholamine. These agents decrease heart rate (chronotopic) and force of contraction (ionotropic) (β_1 effect) and also block the sympathetic stimulation of kidney renin release (β_2 effect).

β-blockers are classified into the following groups based on their structure.

1. **Non-selective β-blockers:** Propranolol, 4-hydroxypropranolol.

2. **Selective β_1 blockers:** Metoprolol, atenolol.

3. **Mixed α/β blockers:** Labetalol, carvedilol.

2.15 SAR OF BETA BLOCKERS

Aryl oxypropanolamine

Most of the β-blockers are similar to β agonist and are in a chemical class of aryloxypropanolamines, only the catechol ring is substituted by different rings to enhance the antagonist activity. Substituting the 3'4' di-hydroxyl group by two chlorine groups leads to dichloroisoproterenol. Unfortunately dichloroisoproterenol has a poor antagonist activity but having good agonist activity.

Dichloroisoproterenol

Catechol group has been replaced by naphthalene to give compounds like pronethnolol. It was a weak antagonist and was withdrawn from clinical testing because of its tendency of forming tumors (mice).

Pronethnolol

An assumption is made that oxymethylene bridge (O-CH$_2$-) group is responsible for the potent antagonist activity, and the side chain has been moved from C$_2$ of the naphthyl group to the C$_1$ position. It has been introduced in between the aromatic ring and ethylamino side chain to give more potent β blockers. For example, propranolol.

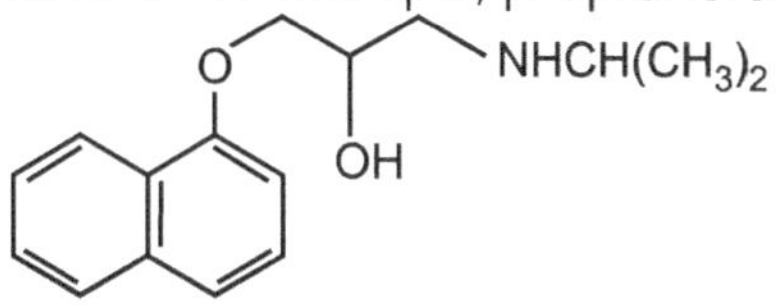

Propranolol

However, most of the drugs containing O-CH$_2$- group are β-agonist. The presence of para substituent on the aromatic ring along with the absence of meta substituent give β$_1$ selective antagonist. e.g. Practolol (cabonamide). Sotalol (Methylsulphonamide).

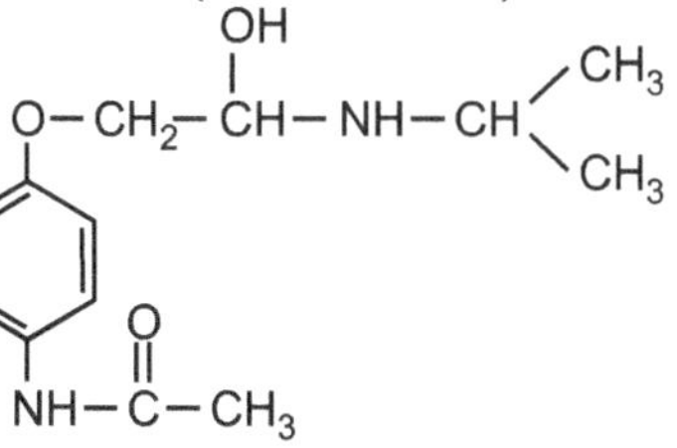

Practolol 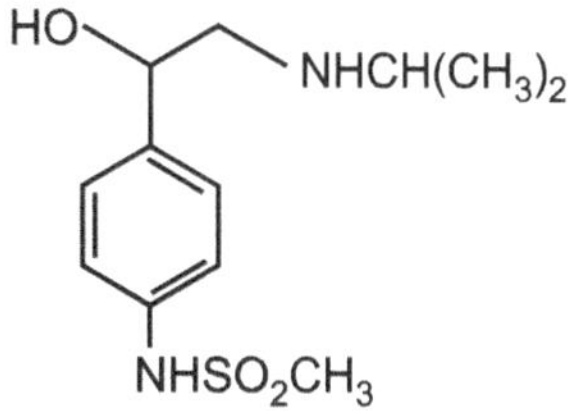　　　　　　　　　　　　　　　**Sotalol**

The bulky aliphatic groups such as tertiary butyl and isopropyl groups (which gives an optimal basicity or nucleophilicity to the amine group for receptor activity) are normally found on the amino functional group of the oxypropanololamine β-receptor antagonist.

B-blockers show high stereoselectivity and for the optimal activity the carbon of the side chain possessing hydroxyl group must be in (S)-configuration. e.g. Timolol, levobunolol.

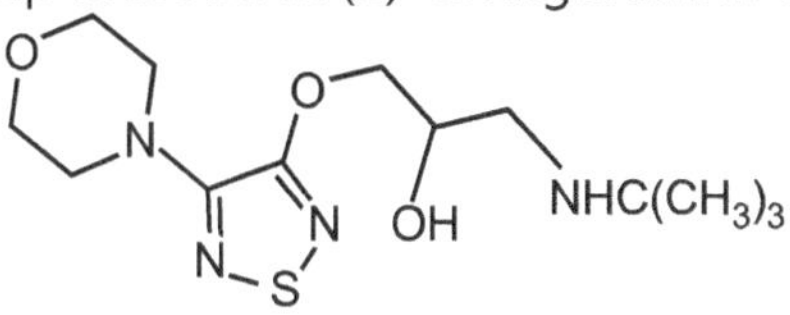

Timolol

2.15.1 Propranolol

Chemically, it is 1-(-isopropylamino)-3-(-1-napthloxy)-2-propranol. It belongs to the class of aryl oxypropranolol amine. It is a non-selective β$_1$ and β$_2$-blocker. Its (S)-isomer is more potent. It has structural similarities as pronethalol (OCH$_3$- bridge between aromatic and ethylamino side chain). It has relatively high lipid solubility and allow distribution to the CNS. One of the metabolite is 4-hydroxypropranolol which shows a potent β-antagonist because of his half life, single dose from 3-4 hours to 5-6 hours.

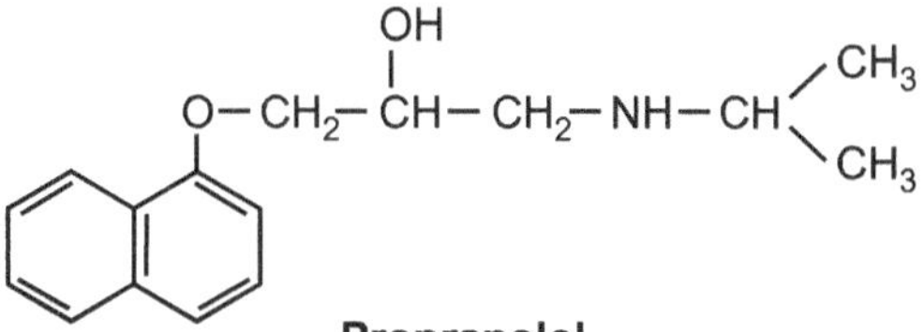

Propranolol

Synthesis: It can be synthesized from naphthol and epichlorohydrin in the presence of hydrochloric acid.

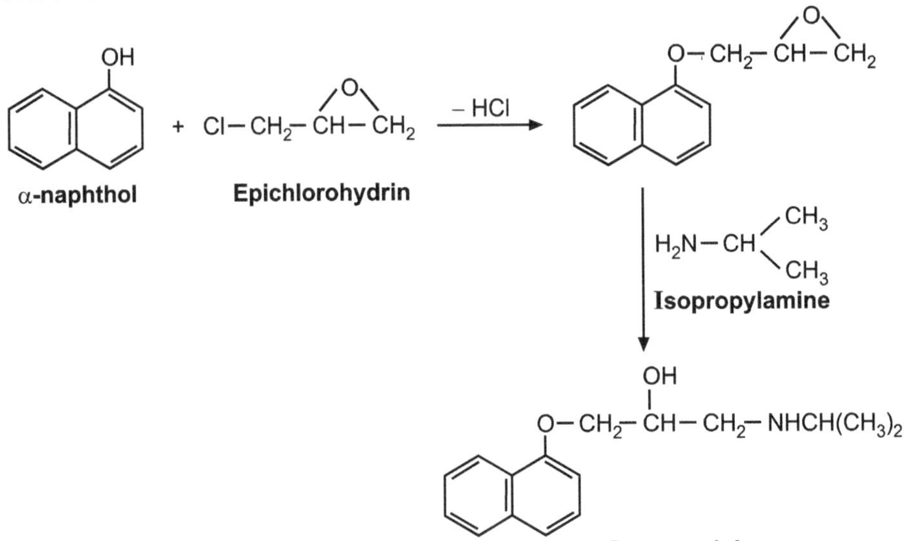

Propranolol

Uses: In the treatment of hypertension, cardiac arrhythmia, angina pectoris, myocardial infarction.

2.15.2 Metibranolol

A beta-adrenergic antagonist effective for both beta-1 and beta-2 receptors. Chemically, it is 4-{[-2-hydroxy-3-(isopropylamino)propyl]oxy}-2,3,6-trimethylphenyl acetate. It is a non-selective β-blocker and metabolised into desacetylmetipranolol.

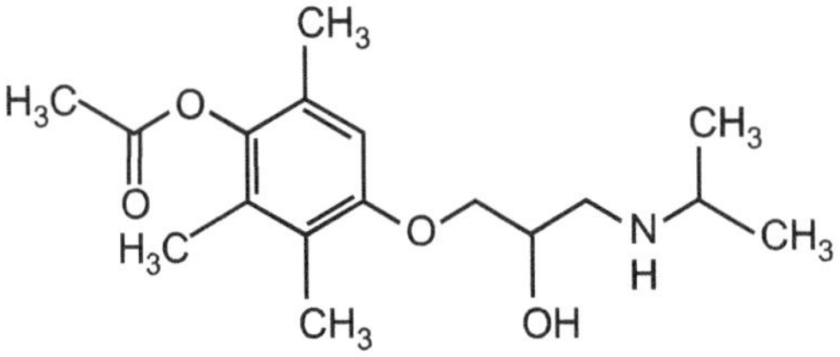

Metibranolol

Uses: It is used as an antiarrhythmic, antihypertensive, and antiglaucoma agent.

2.15.3 Atenolol

Chemically atenolol (R S)-2-[4-(2-Hydroxy-3-isopropylaminopropoxy)-phenyl]- acetamid) is a chiral drug from the group of the selective β_1- adrenoreceptor blockers.

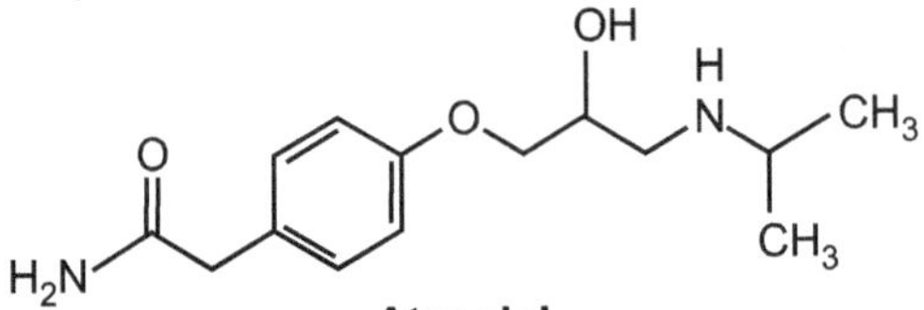

Atenolol

It has low lipid solubility and does not cross blood brain barrier. Thus it has a very less CNS side effects.

Synthesis:

Epichlorohydrin　　　　**2-[4-(2-oxiranylmethoxy) phenyl]acetamide**

Atenolol

Uses: In the treatment of hypertension, angina, myocardial infarction and tachycardia.

2.15.4 Betaxolol

A cardioselective beta-1-adrenergic antagonist with no partial agonist activity. Chemically, it is 1-{4-[2-(cyclopropylmethoxy) ethyl]-phenoxy}-3-(isopropylamino) propan-2-ol. It is a selective β-blocker and shows more affinity towards β_1-receptor.

Betaxolol

Mechanism of Action:

Betaxolol selectively blocks catecholamine stimulation of beta-1-adrenergic receptors in the heart and vascular smooth muscle. This results in a reduction of heart rate, cardiac output, systolic and diastolic blood pressure, and possibly reflex orthostatic hypotension. Betaxolol can also competitively block beta-2-adrenergic responses in the bronchial and vascular smooth muscles, causing bronchospasm.

Uses: In hypertension and glaucoma.

2.15.5 Bisoprolol

Bisoprolol is a cardioselective β_1-adrenergic blocking agent used for secondary prevention of myocardial infarction (MI), heart failure, angina pectoris and mild to moderate hypertension. Bisoprolol is structurally similar to metoprolol, acebutolol and atenolol in that it has two substituents in the *para* position of the benzene ring. The β_1-selectivity of these agents is thought to be due in part to the large substituents in the *para* position. It also shows little activity against β_2-adrenergic receptors of the lungs and vascular smooth muscle. Bisoprolol possesses a single chiral centre and is administered as a racemic mixture. Only *l*-bisoprolol exhibits significant β-blocking activity. Chemically, it is 1-{4-[(2-isopropoxyethoxy) methyl]phenoxy}-3-(isopropylamino)propan-2-ol.

Bisoprolol

Uses: To treat hypertension, heart attacks and kidney problems.

2.15.6 Esmolol

Esmolol (trade name Brevibloc) is a cardioselective β_1 receptor blocker with rapid onset, a very short duration of action, and no significant intrinsic sympathomimetic or membrane stabilizing activity at therapeutic dosages. Chemically it is methyl (RS)-3-{4-[2-hydroxy-3-(propan-2-ylamino)propoxy]phenyl}propanoate. It is short acting β-blocker with rapid onset of action.

Esmolol

Uses: Controlling of heart rate during surgery in operation.

2.15.7 Metoprolol

Chemically, it is 1-[4-(2-Methoxyethyl)phenoxy]-3-[(propan-2-yl)amino]propan-2-ol. It is a selective β_1-blocker. It is lipophilic with intrinsic sympathomimetic activity. It reduces heart rate, heart contractility and blood pressure.

Metoprolol

Uses: In angina pectoris, myocardial infarction and hypertension. Also used in diabetic patients.

2.15.8 Labetalol

Chemically it is 2-hydroxy-5-[1-hydroxy-2-[(4-phenylbutan-2-yl)amino]ethyl] benzamide. It is having both α and β adrenergic blocking activity. In short term it can be used to reduce systemic vascular resistance whereas in long term it reduces the cardiac output.

Labetalol

Uses: Used for the management of hypertension emergencies.

2.15.9 Carvedilol

Carvedilol is a non-selective beta blocker indicated in the treatment of mild to moderate congestive heart failure (CHF). It blocks beta-1 and beta-2 adrenergic receptors as well as the alpha-1 adrenergic receptors. Chemically, it is [3-(9H-carbazol-4-yloxy)-2-hydroxypropyl] [2-(2-methoxyphenoxy)ethyl]amine.

Carvedilol

Uses: To treat congestive heart failure, hypertension.

QUESTIONS

1. Outline the biosynthesis and metabolism of noradraniline.

2. What is adrenergic agonist? Show the principle routes of biosynthesis and metabolism of adrenergic neurotransmitters.

3. Give an account on chemistry and biological activity of adrenergic blocking agent.

4. What are sympathomimetic agents? Discuss their classification and SAR. Give the synthesis of naphazoline.

5. What are adrenergic blocking agents? Give the structures of phenoxybenzamine, prazosin, phentolamine, propranolol, metaprolol and mention their therapeutic applications. Describe the synthesis of propranolol.

6. Write the structure and specific uses for the following.

    (a) Omeprazole

    (b) Pyridostigmine

    (c) Nalorphine

    (d) Propranolol

    (e) Methoxyflurane

7. Outline the synthesis and uses of Propranolol and Dicyclomie.

8. Outline the synthesis and uses of Phenoxybenzamine and Propranolol.

9. Give the SAR of directly acting sympathomimetics.

10. Write a detailed note on adrenergic receptors.

11. Write the examples of sympathomimetic agents and mention their specific uses. Give the synthesis of naphazoline.

12. What are neurotransmitters? Give examples.

13. What are neuronal blocking agents?

14. Name the adrenergic receptors and give their distribution in the body.

15. Give therapeutic uses of beta blockers.

Unit ... 3

CHOLINERGIC DRUGS AND RELATED AGENTS

♦ LEARNING OBJECTIVES ♦

After completing this unit, reader should be able to understand:

❖ To study the difference between central nervous system and peripheral nervous system.

❖ To learn the biosynthesis, metabolism, storage and release of acetylcholine.

❖ To learn about cholinergic receptors and their location.

❖ To learn various para-sympathomimietic and para-sympatholytic agents.

❖ To study synthesis of some selected cholinergic drugs.

3.1 NEUROTRANSMITTERS (NT)

A neurotransmitter is a chemical messenger used by neurons to communicate in one direction with other neurons. Communication between neurons means recognition of the acceptor for a specific chemical messenger. They are synthesized primarily in the nerve terminals stored in vesicles of nerve terminals and are released into electrocellular space using Ca^{2+}.

All neurotransmitters are synthesized at the axon terminals and stored in synaptic vesicles. These synaptic vesicles release neurotransmitter when the presynaptic neuron electrical properties change sufficiently (i.e. arrival of an action potential). Neurotransmitters are released from the vesicles into a tiny space between neurons called the synapse. A bit of released neurotransmitter diffuses across the synaptic space and binds to receptors on the adjacent neuron, the whole process takes about one millisecond. When an neurotransmitter binds to an acceptor on another neuron, ion-channels open and ions move in or out of that neuron. This causes a net change in the electrical properties (membrane potential of that neuron and determines its activity). The change may be inhibitory or excitatory and is determined by the receptor on the post-synaptic neuron.

3.2 CHOLINERGIC NEUROTRANSMITTERS

Acetylcholine is a neurotransmitter parasympathetic nervous system. Acetylcholine (ACh) is the chemical transmitter at both pre and postganglionic synapses in the parasympathetic system. Ach is also the neurotransmitter at sympathetic preganglionic synapses, some sympathetic of postganglionic synapses, the neuromuscular junction (somatic nervous system), and at some sites in the CNS. Acetylcholine is the most widespread autonomic transmitter present in the body. Cholinergic transmission can occur through muscarinic (G protein-coupled) or nicotinic (ionotropic) receptors and the muscarinic receptor is terminated by the action of cholinesterases.

3.3 SYNTHESIS OF ACETYLCHOLINE (ACh)

The major steps in the synthesis of acetylcholine are illustrated in the figure below. Acetylcholine was also one of the first neurotransmitters identified due to its presence in the peripheral nervous system. Acetylcholine is the neurotransmitter at all the motor targeted synapses in the somatic branch of the peripheral nervous system. In addition, it is the neurotransmitter at the parasympathetic postganglionic-target synapses in the autonomic nervous system. (Recall that norepinephrine is the neurotransmitter at the corresponding sympathetic synapses.) In the central nervous system, acetylcholine is best known for its role in memory and learning. For example, Alzheimer's disease is associated with a break down in acetylcholine neurons. Acetylcholine is synthesized locally in the choleric nerve ending by the following pathway:

- An amino acid Serine is the precursor for the synthesis of acetylcholine. Serine undergoes decarboxylation in the presence of serine decarboxylase to choline.
- Choline is actively taken up by the axonal membrane by a Na^+, choline cotransporter and acetylated with the help of ATP and coenzyme-A enzyme choline acetyl transferase present in the axoplasm.
- Most of the ACh is stored in ionic solution within small synaptic vesicles, but some free Ca^{2+} also present in the cytoplasm of cholinergic terminals. Active transport of ACh into synaptic vesicles is affected by another carrier.

Release of ACh:

When Ca^{2+} ion concentration is high in intracellular with cell membrane and release of this content into the synaptic cleft.

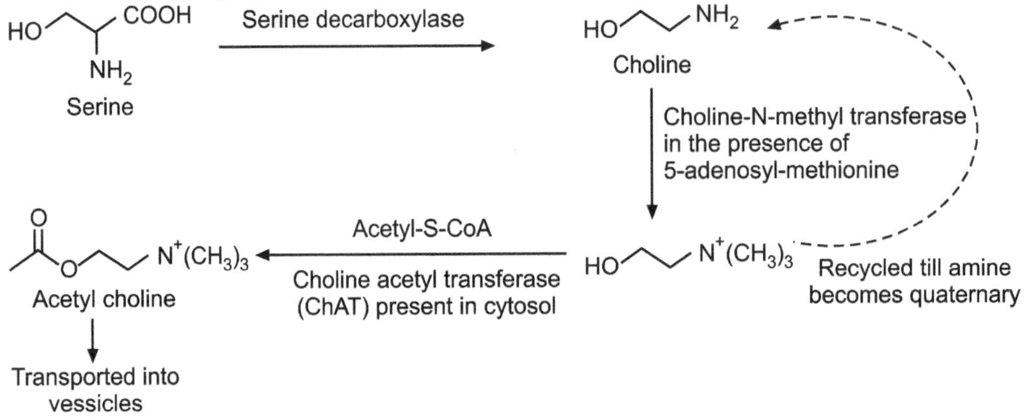

HO COOH
NH₂
Serine
Serine decarboxylase
HO NH₂
Choline
Choline-N-methyl transferase in the presence of 5-adenosyl-methionine
HO N⁺(CH₃)₃
Recycled till amine becomes quaternary
Acetyl-S-CoA
Choline acetyl transferase (ChAT) present in cytosol
N⁺(CH₃)₃
Acetyl choline
Transported into vessicles

Degradation of ACh:

Acetyl cholinesterase cleavages ACh to choline and acetate.

3.4 CHOLINERGIC RECEPTORS

The acetylcholine (ACh) receptor, at the neuromuscular junction, is a neurotransmitter-gated ion channel that has been fine-tuned through evolution to transduce a chemical signal into an electrical signal with maximum efficiency and speed. It is composed from three similar and two identical polypeptide chains, arranged in a ring around a narrow membrane pore. Central to the design of this assembly is a hydrophobic gate in the pore, more than 50 A° away from sites in the extracellular domain where ACh binds.

There are two main types of cholinergic receptor.

- Nicotinic cholinergic receptor.
- Muscarinic cholinergic receptor.

Nicotinic and muscarinic ACh receptors are named after two substances which bind to those receptor subtypes. Nicotine binds to nicotinic, but not muscarinic ACh receptors. Muscarinic receptors are named after Muscarine, found in some species of mushroom.

Nicotinic receptors, when ACh interacts with a nicotinic ACh receptor, it opens a Na^+ channel and Na^+ ions flow into the membrane. This causes a depolarization, and results in an EPSP. Thus, ACh is excitatory on skeletal muscle. The electrical response is fast, and short lived. Nicotinic receptors are mainly located in CNS automatic ganglia and neuromuscular junction (NMJ).

Muscarinic receptors are located primarily on autonomic effector cells in heart blood vessels, eye, smooth muscles and gland of gastrointestinal, respiratory and urinary tracts, sweat glands and in the CNS.

They are classified into sub-types according to their molecular structure, signal transduction, and ligand affinity in M_1, M_2, M_3, M_4, M_5.

In M_1, M_2 and M_4 type of muscarinic receptors, ACh acts by stimulating or activating Gq protein and release phospholipase C, the G-protein activates channels or enzymes indirectly and responses are diverse, slower, and longer-lived.

3.5 PARASYMPATHOMIMETIC (PSM) AGENTS

Compounds that mimic the action of ACh at parasympathetic system are called as cholinergic parasymathomimetic agents. Thus these drugs stimulate the effect of cells innervated by postganglionic parasympathetic cholinergic nerves. They are classified as directly acting and indirectly acting cholinergics.

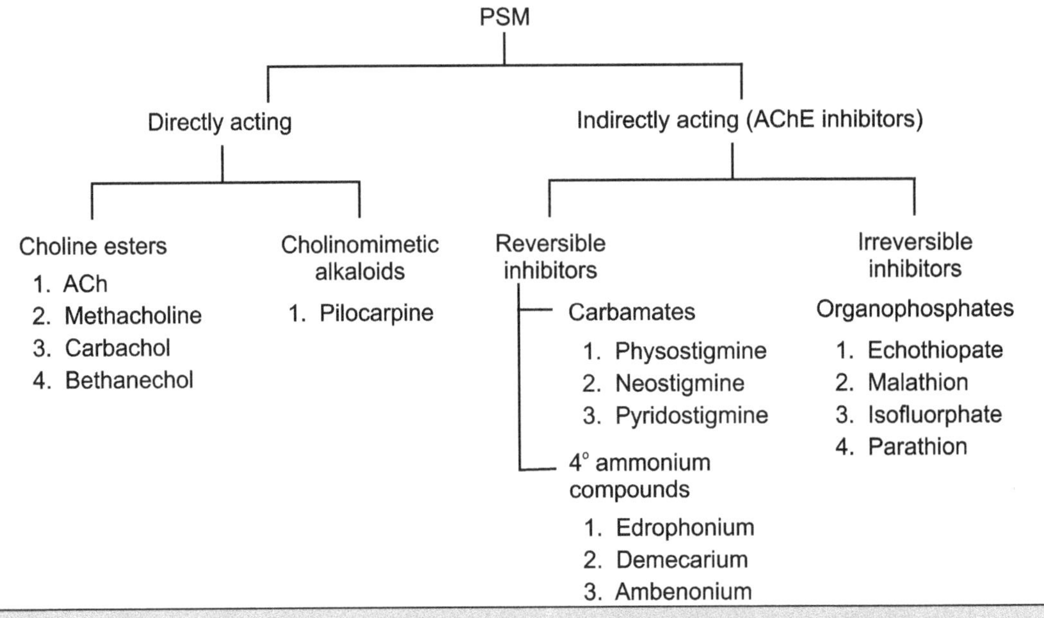

3.6 SAR OF PARASYMPATHOMIMETIC / CHOLINERGIC AGONIST

➤ Acetylcholine is the ester of choline, is a quaternary ammonium compound which possess a cationic (positively charged) part joined by a two carbon chain to an ester group.

➤ **Modification of the Quaternary Ammonium Group:**

• The quaternary ammonium group is essential for intrinsic activity and contribute to the affinity of the molecule for the receptors, partially through the binding energy and partially because of its action as a detecting group.

• The trimethyl ammonium group is essential for the optimal functional activity. (Although some exceptions which show muscarinic activity. e.g. pilocarpine, nicotine).

• Replacement of Nitrogen (N) by other atoms like Sulphur (S), Arsenic (As) or Selenium (Se) leads to decrease into the activity.

Pilocarpine

• Placement of primary, secondary or tertiary amine leads to decrease the activity.

➤ **Modification of Ester Group:**
- The ester group of ACh contributes to the binding of the compound to the muscarinic receptors.
- Replacement of ethyl group or bulky alkyl group leads to inactive compounds.
- Ester of higher aromatic acids possesses cholinergic antagonist activity. e.g. Bethanechol, Methancholine.

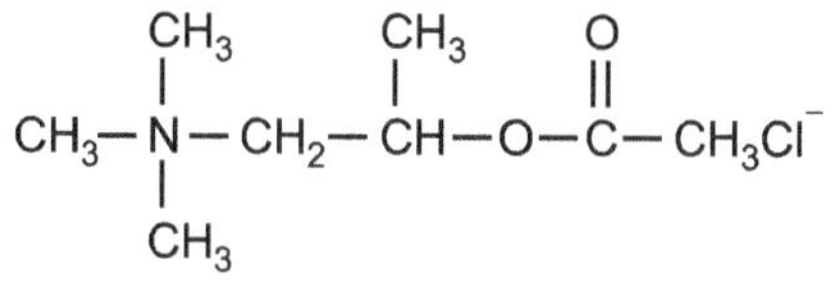

$$CH_3-\overset{\overset{\displaystyle CH_3}{|}}{\underset{\underset{\displaystyle CH_3}{|}}{N}}-CH_2-\overset{\overset{\displaystyle CH_3}{|}}{CH}-O-\overset{\overset{\displaystyle O}{||}}{C}-CH_3Cl^{-} \qquad \text{Methacholine} - Cl^{-}$$

$$CH_3-\overset{\overset{\displaystyle CH_3}{|}}{\underset{\underset{\displaystyle CH_3}{|}}{N}}-CH_2-\overset{\overset{\displaystyle CH_3}{|}}{CH}-O-\overset{\overset{\displaystyle O}{||}}{C}-NH_2Cl^{-} \qquad \text{Bethanechol} - Cl^{-}$$

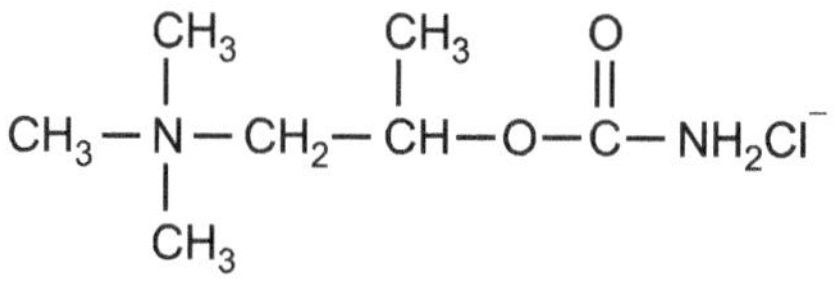

- NH_2 group can be introduced in place of CH_3. It is more stable than carboxylate ester towards hydrolysis.

➤ **Modification of Ethylene Bridge:**
- For maximum muscarinic activity there should not be more than four atoms in between the quaternary ammonium group and ester molecule. A series of N-alkyl trimethyl ammonium salts shows optimum muscarinic activity.
- The methyl ester is rapidly hydrolysed by cholinesterase to choline and acetic acid. To reduce susceptibility to hydrolysis, carbamate esters of choline were synthesised and found to be more stable than carboxylated esters. E.g. Neostigmine

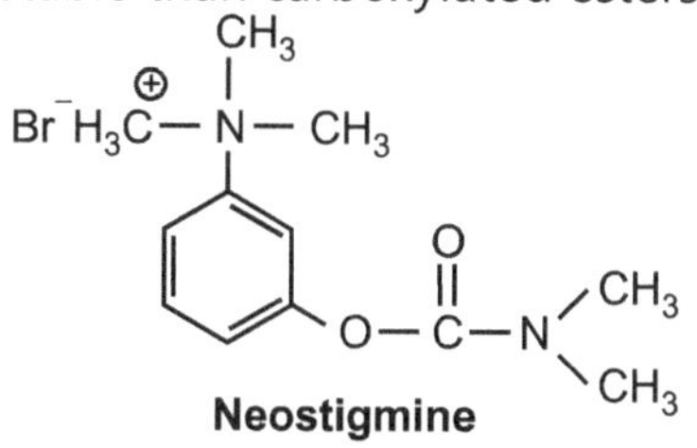

Neostigmine

- Placement of α-substitution in choline moiety results in a reduction of both muscarinic and nicotinic activity.
- Substitution at β-position leads to compounds with decrease in activity. E.g. methacholine.
- Replacement of ester group with ether or ketone produces chemically stable and potent compounds. E.g. Muscarine, pilocarpine.

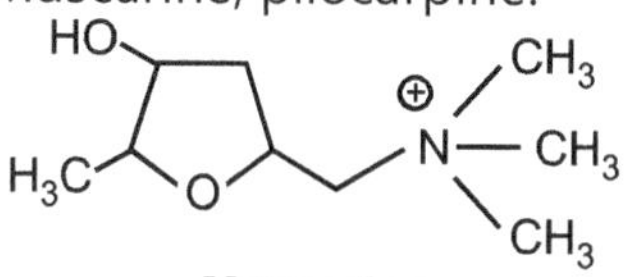

Muscarine

Directly Acting Cholinergic Drugs:

The directly acting cholinomimetic drugs are divided on the basis of their chemical structures into:

- Choline esters and
- Cholinomimetic alkaloids

3.7 CHOLINE ESTERS

Choline esters are synthetic derivatives of choline. They stimulate muscarinic receptors affecting the cardiac muscle, smooth muscle, exocrine glands and the eye. Choline esters are lipid insoluble and do not readily enter the CNS (effects occur primarily in the periphery). They are highly resistant to being destroyed by acetylcholinesterase (AChE). The choline esters differ in their relative sensitivity to hydrolysis and in their relative nicotinic and muscarinic effects. Thus, methacholine, while still susceptible to hydrolysis, is much more stable than ACh, and carbachol and bethanechol are resistant to hydrolysis by AChE. Carbachol has a high level of nicotinic activity, methacholine with little nicotinic activity, and bethanechol essentially of no nicotinic activity.

3.7.1 Bethanechol

- Bethanechol is a synthetic derivative of choline.
- Bethanechol is a carbomic ester of β-methylcholine.
- It is not rapidly hydrolysed by acetycholinesterase and has strong muscarinic actions but little nicotinic actions.
- The presence of CH_3 gives prolonged activity due to steric hindrance.
- It produces smooth muscle contractions. It is not well absorbed from GI tract (large doses required). It can be given subcutaneously but not by IM or IV routes because of severe adverse effects.
- It is used in the relief of urinary retention and abdominal distention after surgery.

$$(CH_3)_3\overset{+}{N}-CH_2-\underset{\underset{CH_3}{|}}{CHO}-\overset{\overset{O}{\|}}{C}-NH_2$$

Bethanechol

3.7.2 Carbachol

- Carbachol is an ester of carbamic acid. In carbachol, the terminal methyl group of acetylcholine is replaced by amino ($-NH_2$) group.
- It possesses both muscarinic as well as nicotinic properties by cholinergic receptor stimulation.
- Carbachol is a poor substrate for acetyl choline esterase and therefore is not readily hydrolysed than acetyl choline.

- The presence of carbonyl group in carbachol decreases the electrophilicity and form resonance structures more easily then ACh. Thus less susceptible to hydrolysis, more stable in aqueous solution.
- Carbachol has a high level of nicotinic activity than compared with methacholine.
- It reduces intraocular pressure. Carbachol is used to induce miosis (pupil constriction) and relieve intraocular pressure of glaucoma.

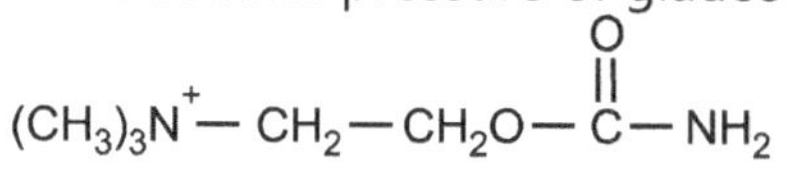

$$(CH_3)_3\overset{+}{N}-CH_2-CH_2O-\overset{\overset{\displaystyle O}{\|}}{C}-NH_2$$

Carbamylcholine (Carbachol)

Synthesis:

It can be prepared by treating phosgene with ethylene chlorohydrin to form chloroethylchlorofornate. Chloroethylchloroformate then treated in the presence of ammonia and ether gives urethane which is then heated with trimethylamine to yield carbachol.

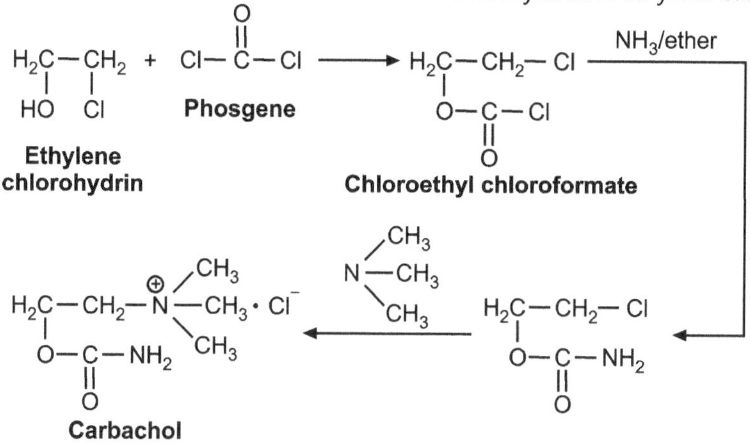

Carbachol

3.7.3 Methacholine

- Methacholine is available as methacholine chloride. Chemically methacholine is 2-acetoxypropyltrimethyl ammonium chloride.
- Methacholine, is still susceptible to hydrolysis but much more stable than ACh, and carbachol and bethanechol which are resistant to hydrolysis by AChE.
- Methacholine can exist as (S) and (R) enantiomers, but its muscarinic activity resides in the (S) isomer.
- Methacholine was used in the past to control supraventricular tachycardia and is replaced with ectrophonium and other drugs, which are safer.
- Methacholine is also used for diagnosis of belladonna poisoning, for diagnosis of familial dysautonomia, and for diagnosis of bronchial hyper reactivity.

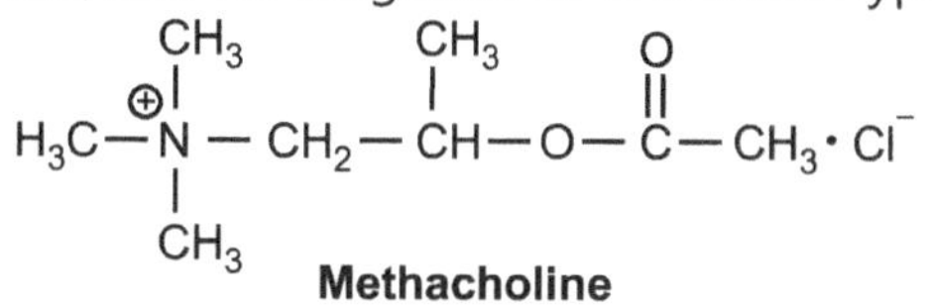

Methacholine

3.8 CHOLINOMIMETIC ALKALOIDS

Muscarine, arecoline, pilocarpine are natural alkaloids. The actions of these alkaloids are similar to that of choline esters and show more CNS side effects. Pilocarpine, muscarine, and oxotremorine are relatively specific for muscarinic acetyl choline receptors,

3.8.1 Pilocarpine

- Pilocarpine is an alkaloid obtained from the dried leaflets of Pilocarpus jaborandi.
- It is available as hydrochloride and nitrate salt. Chemically it is 3-ethyldihydro-4 [(1-methyl-1H-imida zol-5-yl)-methyl] furan-2(3H)-one.
- It binds to muscarinic receptor as an non-selective agonist.
- It cannot penetrate the membrane because of bulky substituents but penetrate the eye membrane when applied topically.
- These drugs (essentially only pilocarpine) are used in the treatment of glaucoma.

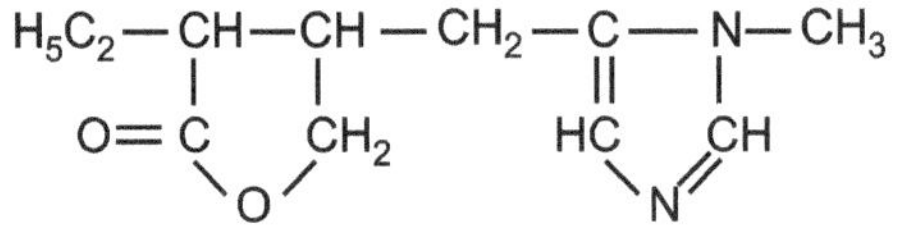

$$H_5C_2-CH-CH-CH_2-C-N-CH_3$$

Pilocarpine

3.9 INDIRECTLY ACTING CHOLINERGIC DRUGS (ACETYLCHOLINESTERASE INHIBITORS)

These drugs inhibit the cholineseterase enzymes and thereby stimulate the production of acetylcholine. It terminates the biological activity of acetylcholine by hydrolysing acetylcholine into acetic acid and choline molecule.

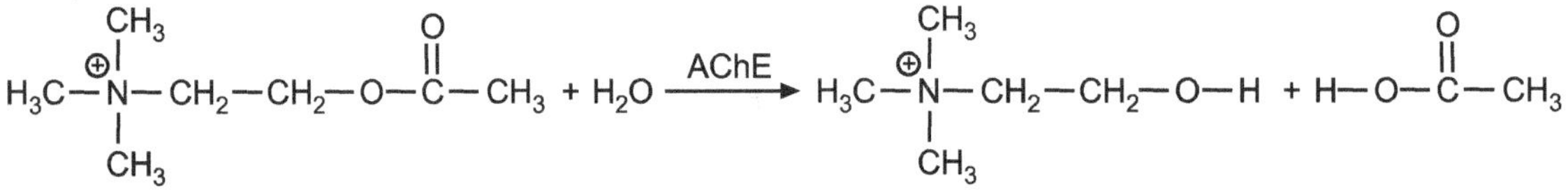

$$H_3C-\overset{\oplus}{N}(CH_3)-CH_2-CH_2-O-\overset{O}{C}-CH_3 + H_2O \xrightarrow{AChE} H_3C-\overset{\oplus}{N}(CH_3)-CH_2-CH_2-O-H + H-O-\overset{O}{C}-CH_3$$

Acetyl choline   **Choline molecule**   **Acetic acid**

It is found in RBCs in the brain and other nerve tissue. It is present in high concentration on the presynaptic sites, postsynaptic sites and at the motor nerve end of the cholinergic neurons. Acetylcholinesterase has three important sites, the anionic, cationic and esteratic sites.

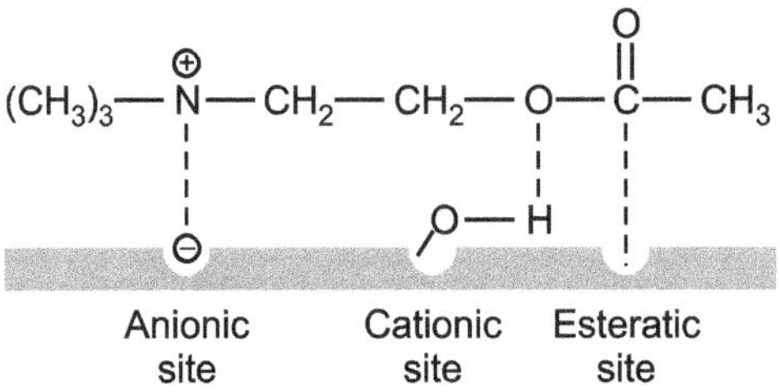

$$(CH_3)_3-\overset{\oplus}{N}-CH_2-CH_2-O-\overset{O}{C}-CH_3$$

Anionic   Cationic   Esteratic
site   site   site

The anionic site of enzyme binds with the quaternary nitrogen of the ACh through ionic and hydrophobic forces. At this site the Y-carboxylate group of the glutamic acid residue acts as a strong nucleophile then attack on the C-carbon of carbonyl moiety to form tetrahedral intermediate. This intermediate collapses to form choline molecule. The hydroxyl group binds at the cationic site. The esteratic site consists of two imidazole rings from histidine and serine moieties (Im_1 and Im_2). The imidazole group of Im_1 accepts proton from serine and hydroxyl from tyrosine site to bind with the ether oxygen of acetylcholine. Choline molecule forms, undergo dissociation and conformational changes. In presence of second imidazole ring which catalyses hydrolysis of acetylated serine to give acetic acid and serine residue.

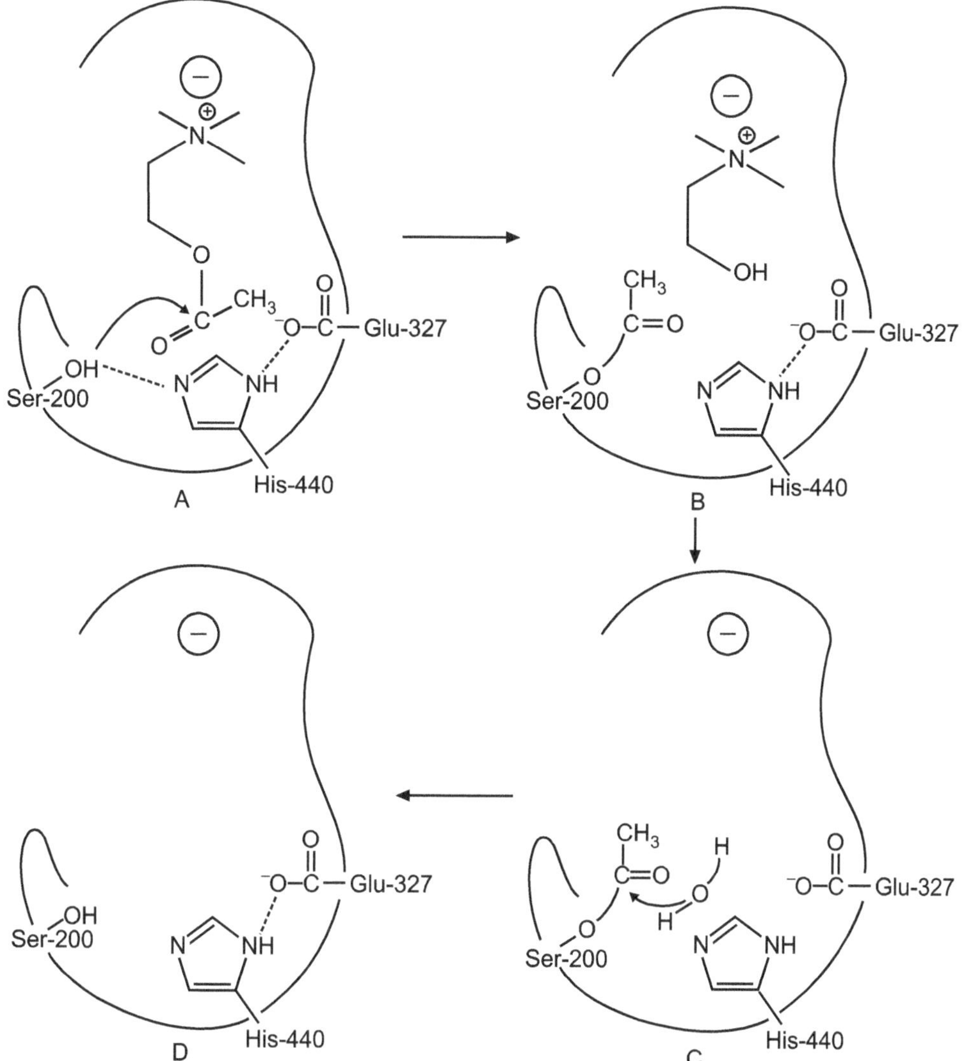

Fig. 3.1: Mechanism of hydrolysis of ACh by AChE.

(A) ACh-AChE-reversible complex, (B) Acetylation of esteratic site, (C) General base-catalysed hydrolysis of acetylated enzyme, (D) Free enzyme

Acetylcholinesterase inhibitors have been used clinically in the treatment of myasthenia gravis. They are also employed to treat glaucoma and more recently in Alzheimer's disease.

3.10 CLASSIFICATION OF ANTI-CHOLINESTERASES

The anticholinesterases are classified into:

➢　Reversible anti-cholinesterases.

➢　Irreversible anti-cholinesterases.

3.10.1 Reversible Anti-cholinesterases

They were structually resemble to choline esterases and can compete for the binding sites of cholinesterase receptors. Thus it causes inhibition of the enzyme for short duration of time.

3.10.1.1 Physostigmine

➢　Physostigmine, a tertiary amine, is an alkaloid obtained from the *physostigma venenosum*.

➢　Chemically, it is 1, 2, 3, 3α, 8, 8α-hexahydro-1, 3α, 8-trimethyl-pyrrolo [2,3-b] indol-5-methylcarbamate. It is a reversible acetylcholinesterases inhibitor.

➢　Physostigmine reversibly inhibits acetylcholinesterase thus results in potentiation of cholinergic activity. It stimulates muscarinic, nicotinic sites of ANS and nicotinic receptors of neuromuscular junction.

➢　Used in the treatment of Alzheimer's disease, glaucoma and as an antidote during dhatura poisoning.

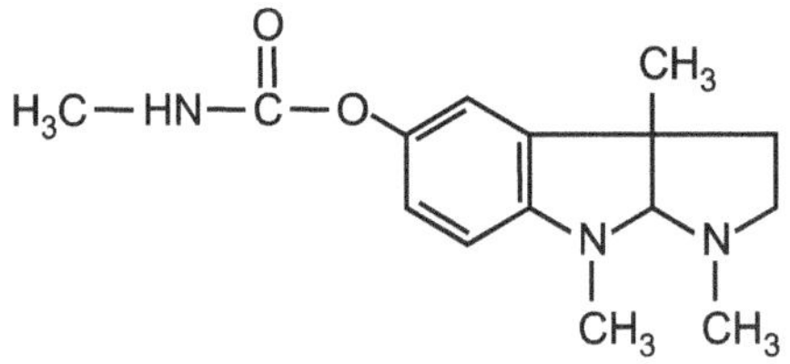

Physostigmine

3.10.1.2 Neostigmine

➢　Chemically, it is 3-{[(Dimethylamino)carbonyl]oxy}-N,N,N-trimethylbenzenaminium. Neostigmine is available as a bromide and methyl sulphate salt It is an reversible acetylcholinesterases inhibitor and can be administered along with atropine.

➢　Used in the treatment of Myasthenia gravis, Ogilvie's syndrome and in case of snake bite.

➢　Neostigmine inhibits both AChE and butylcholineesterase reversibly and potentiates nicotinic and muscarinic effects of acetylcholine.

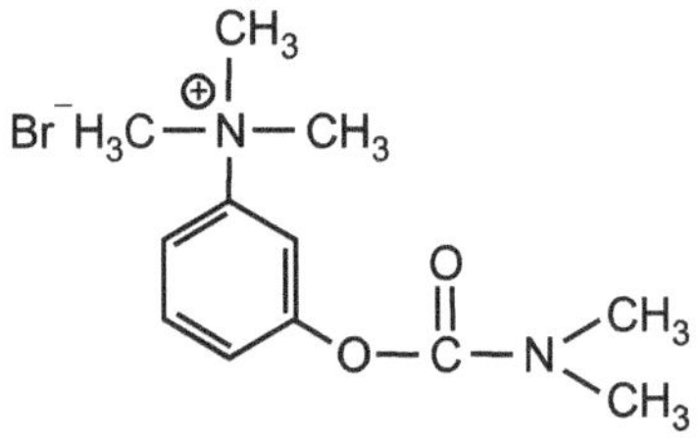

Neostigmine

Synthesis:

It is synthesized from N, N-Dimethylcarbonyl chloride and 3-Hydroxy N, N-dimethylaniline.

N,N-Dimethylcarbonyl chloride

3.10.1.3 Pyridostigmine

- Pyridostigmine is a pyridine analogue of neostigmine.
- Chemically, it is 3-[(dimethylcarbamoyl)oxy]-1-methylpyridinium. It is an reversible acetylcholinesterases inhibitor.
- Pyridostigmine is a potent reversible inhibitor of acetylcholinesterase. By inhibiting the enzyme it permits free transmission of nerve impulses across the neuromuscular junction. It is hydrolyzed by acetylcholinesterase but much more slowly than acetylcholine itself.
- Pyridostigmine intensifies both the nicotinic and muscarinic effects of acetylcholine. It can be given and administered by IV.

Pyridostigmine

3.10.1.4 Edrophonium Chloride

- Edrophonium is available as edrophonium chloride. Chemically, it is N-Ethyl-3-hydroxy-N,N-dimethylbenzenaminium. It is reversible acetylcholinesterases inhibitor.
- It acts by inhibiting competitively the enzyme acetylcholinesterase at the neuromuscular junction.
- Quaternary ammonium compounds inhibit the enzyme reversibly by either binding with the esteratic site or the peripheral anionic site.
- Edrophonium chloride is an anti-AChE agent with a rapid onset but short duration of action. Edrophonium binds reversibly and selectively to the active center; this reversible binding and its rapid renal elimination result in its short duration of action. It has been used in myasthenia gravis.

Edrophonium chloride

3.10.1.5 Tacrine Hydrochloride

➢ Chemically, it is 1,2,3,4-tetrahydroacridin-9-amine. It is reversible inhibitor of acetylcholinesterases.

➢ It has a longer duration of action.

➢ Used in the treatment of Alzheimer's disease and analeptic agent to promote mental awareness.

Tacrine hydrochloride

3.10.1.6 Ambenonium Chloride

➢ Ambenonium occurs as ambenonium chloride. Chemically, it is [oxalylbis(iminoethylene)] bis[(*o*-chlorobenzyl)diethylammonium]dichloride.

➢ It acts by suppressing the activity of acetylcholinesterase by competitive reverse inhibition. It is not hydrolysed by AChE.

➢ Used: to treat myasthenia gravis in patients who do not respond satisfactory to neostigmine or pyridostigmine.

Ambenonium chloride

3.10.2 Irreversible Anti-cholinesterases

These compounds are generally organophosphorus compounds and combined with the esteratic site of cholinesterase and get phosphorylated. The process is slow and produces a long term inhibition of cholinesterases.

3.10.2.1 Isofluorphate

➢ Isofluorphate is an organophosphate compound and chemically it is bis(propan-2-yl) fluorophosphonate.

➢ Isofluorphate irreversibly inhibits cholinesterase, its activity lasts for days or even week.

➢ Used in the treatment of glaucoma.

Isofluorphate

3.10.2.2 Echothiophate Iodide (Phospholine)

➢ Echothiophate is an organophosphate available as echothiophate iodide. Chemically, it is 2-(Diethoxyphosphorylsulfanyl)ethyl-N,N,N-trimethylazanium iodide.

➢ It is a long acting irreversible acetylcholinesterase inhibitor.

➢ It has a short duration of action with rapid onset and elimination of drug. Used in the treatment of glaucoma and as an irreversible cholinesterase.

Ecothiophate iodide

3.10.2.3 Parathion

➢ Parathion is O, O-diethyl O-p-nitrophenyl phosphorothioate. It is an organothiophosphate compound having week anticholinesterase activity.

➢ Used as agricultural insecticide and irreversible cholinesterase.

Parathion

3.10.2.4 Malathion

➢ Malathion is a phosphodithioate ester, chemically 2-[(dimethoxyphosphinothioyl)thio]-butanedioic acid diethyl ester. It is an organophosphate compound and acts as an acetylcholinesterases inhibitor.

➢ Malathion is used extensively for controlling insects on vegetables, fruits, and cereal crops. It is also used for controlling insects affecting man and animals.(e.g. Mosquitoes).

Malathion

3.10.2.5 Pralidoxime

➢ Pralidoxime is an aldoxime and available as pralidoxime chloride. Chemically it is 2-formyl-1-methylpyridinium chloride oxime.

➢ Pralidoxime is a useful antidote for intoxication with cholinesterase inhibitors such as the organophosphates.

Synthesis:

Picolinal is converted into its oxime. The formed oxime is converted to pralidoxime methosulfate with dimethylsulphate, which on treatment with hydrochloric acid forms pralidoxime chloride.

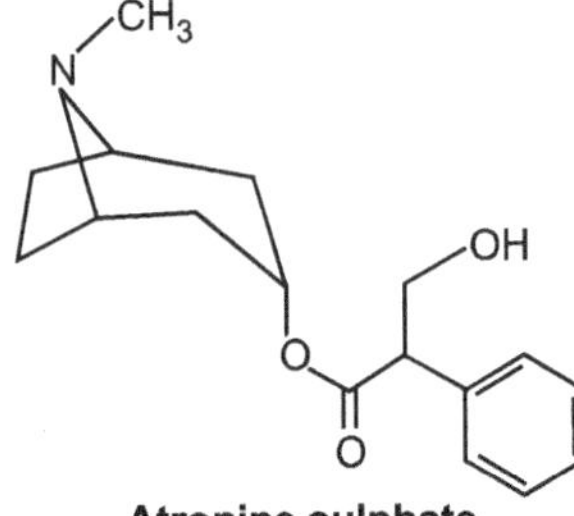

3.11 SOLANACEOUS ALKALOIDS AND ANALOGUES

3.11.1 Atropine Sulphate

- Chemically, it is (8-Methyl-8-azabicyclo[3.2.1]oct-3-yl) 3-hydroxy-2-phenylpropanoate.
- It is an antimuscarinic agent and act by inhibiting the parasympathetic nervous system. It can be administered by IV or IM.
- Hyoscymaine sulphate: It is a tropane alkaloid. 8-methyl-8-azabicyclo[3.2.1]octan-3-yl 3-hydroxy-2-phenylpropanoate.
- It is an antagonist of muscarinic acetylcholine receptor. It blocks the action of acetylcholine at parasympathetic sites.
- Used to treatement of spasm caused by peptic ulcer, irritable bowel syndrome, pancreatitis. Also to treat Parkinson's disease and abnormal respiratory symptoms.

Atropine sulphate

3.11.2 Scopolamine Hydrobromide (Hyoscine)

- Chemically, it is 3-Hydroxy-2-phenylpropionic acid (1R,2R,4S,5S,7α,9S)-9-methyl-3-oxa-9-azatricyclo[3.3.1.02,4]non-7-yl ester.
- It is natural alkaloid and consider to be one of the safe drug.
- Used to treat motion sickness and post-operative nausea- vomiting. It is also given as pre-anestheticdrug. It has an antispasmodic activity.

Hyoscine

3.11.3 Homatropine Hydrobromide

- ➢ Chemically, it is N-Methyl-8-azabicyclo[3.2.1]oct-3-yl) 2-hydroxy-2-phenylacetate.
- ➢ It is an muscarinic antagonist receptor.
- ➢ It is a synthetic alkaloid. It is available as colourless, crystalline and odourless solid. It has a rapid onset of action as compared to atropine and used in mydriasis.
- ➢ Used to treat mydriasis. Also to treat peptic ulcer and gastrointestinal spasm.

3.11.4 Ipratropium Bromide

- ➢ Chemically, it is [8-methyl-8-(1-methylethyl)-8-azoniabicyclo[3.2.1] oct-3-yl] 3-hydroxy-2-phenyl-propanoate.
- ➢ It's a muscarinic antagonist and used to treat the chronic obstructive pulmonary disease (COPD) and asthama COPD.

Synthesis: It is synthesised from acetyl chloride treated with the acid chloride to give compound-1 which subsequently treated with acid chloride to give compound-2. Isopropyl alcohol with an organic acid denture base product was dissolved in dichloromethane, added via acylation of compound 2 to give compound-3. Compound-3 to give Compound-4 alcoholysis reaction. 4-bromo-methyl compound to give compound-5 i.e. ipratropium bromide.

3.12 SYNTHETIC CHOLINERGIC BLOCKING AGENTS

3.12.1 Tropicamide

➤ Chemically, it is N-ethyl-3-hydroxy-2-phenyl-N-(pyridin-4-ylmethyl)propanamide. It is an anticholinergic drug and produces short acting mydriasis.

➤ Used as an mydriatic agent.

Tropicamide

3.12.2 Cyclopentolate Hydrochloride

➤ Chemically, it is 2-(dimethylamino) ethyl (1-hydroxycyclopentyl) (phenyl) acetate. It is a muscarinic antagonist. It dilates the eye by blocking the muscarinic receptors. It can be used as a substitute of atropine.

➤ Used as an mydriatic agent. Also used to treat keratitis, choroiditis and iritis.

Cyclopentolate hydrochloride

3.12.3 Clidinium Bromide

➤ Chemically, it is 3-[(2-hydroxy-2,2-diphenylacetyl)oxy]-1-methyl-1-azabicyclo[2.2.2]octan-1-ium bromide. It is an anticholinergic muscarinic antagonist.

➤ Used in the treatment of peptic ulcer, hyperchlorhydria, and ulcerative or spastic-colon.

Clidinium bromide

3.12.4 Dicyclomine Hydrochloride

➤ Chemically, it is 2-(Diethylamino)ethyl 1-cyclohexylcyclohexane-1-carboxylate. It is an anticholinergic, antispasmodic agent and a smooth muscle relaxant in the GI and urinary tract.

➤ Used to treat renal, intestinal, irritable bowel and dysmenorrhoea.

Dicyclomine hydrochloride

Synthesis:

Cyclohexylnitrile on alkylation with 1,5-dibromopentane gives a cyclohexane intermediate which on hydrolysis gives acid. It is then esterified with N,N-diethylamino ethanol to get dicyclomine.

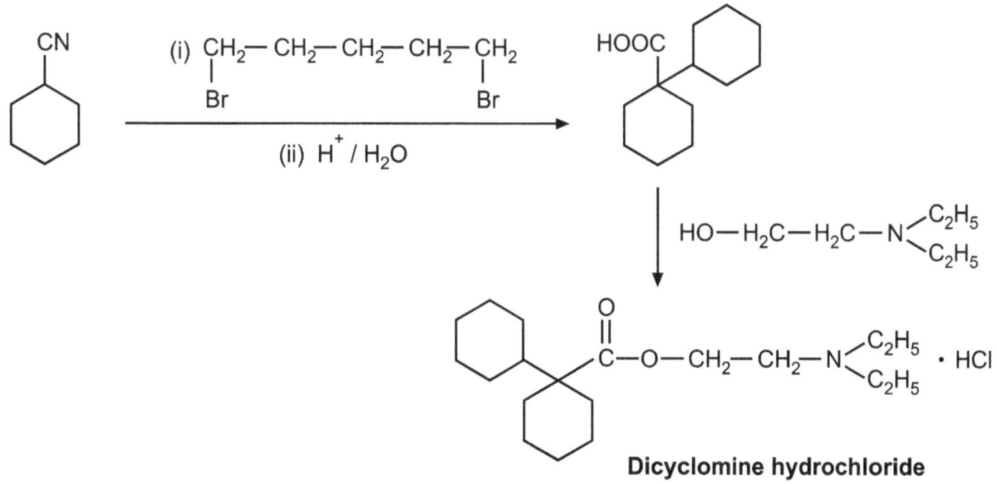

Dicyclomine hydrochloride

3.12.5 Glycopyrrolate

➢ Chemically, glycopyrrolate is 3-[2-Cyclopentyl(hydroxy)phenylacetoxy]-1,1-dimethylpyrrolidinium bromide.

➢ It is an muscarinic antagonist. It can be administered orally and by IV route.

➢ Used as anticholinergic, and antispasmodic agent in gastrointestinal spasm.

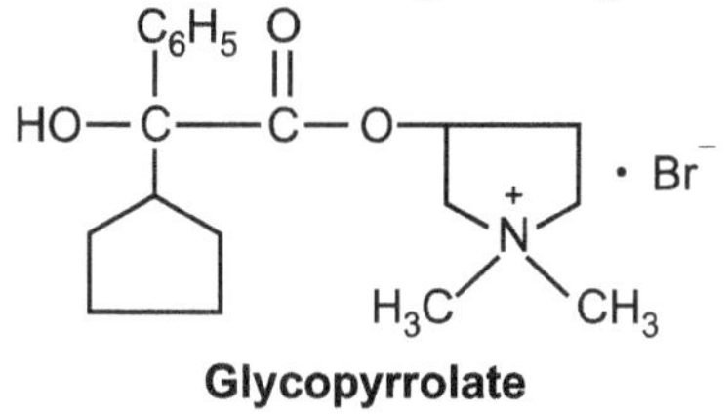

Glycopyrrolate

3.12.6 Methantheline Bromide

➢ Chemically, it is N, N-diethyl-N-methyl-2-[(9H-xanthen-9-ylcarbonyl)oxy]-ethanaminium. It is an anti-muscarinic and act on the postganglionic cholinergic nerve.

➢ Used to relive spasms or cramps of the stomach, intestine and bladder. Also used to treat peptic ulcer.

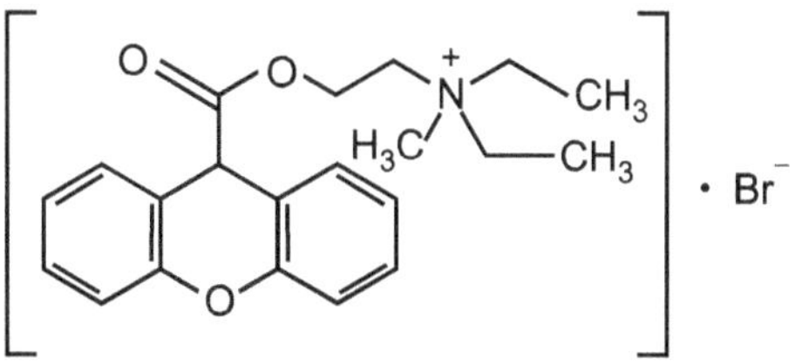

Methantheline bromide

3.12.7 Propantheline Bromide

➤ Chemically, 3-[2-Cyclopentyl(hydroxy)phenylacetoxy]-1,1-dimethylpyrrolidinium bromide. It is a muscarinic antagonist and have poor ability to cross the blood-brain-barrier.

➤ Used to reduce excessive saliva. It has high ratio of ganglionic blocking activity to muscarinic activity. It is used as antispasmodic and in the treatment of peptic ulcers.

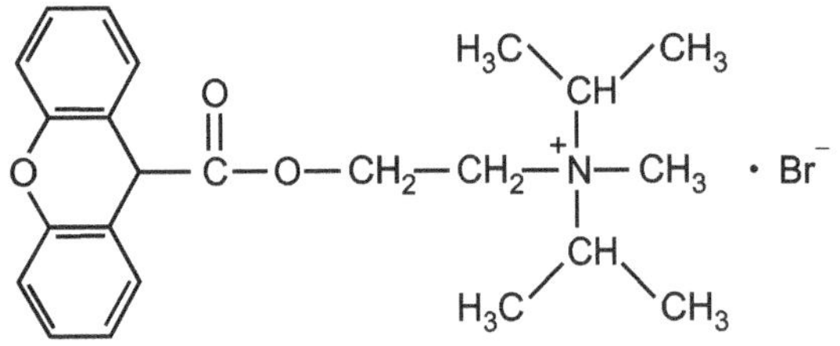

Propantheline bromide

3.12.8 Benztropine Mesylate

➤ Chemically, it is 3-(Diphenylmethoxy)-8-methyl-8-azabicyclo[3.2.1]octane. It is an anticholinergic drug.

➤ Used in the treatment of Parkinson's disease. As an antihistaminic and local anaesthetic.

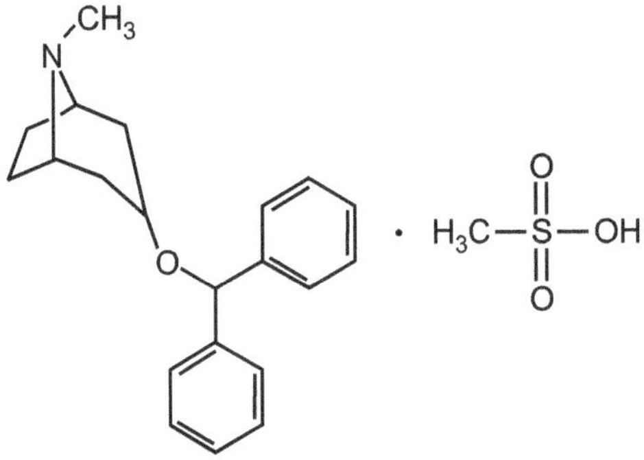

Benztropine mesylate

3.12.9 Orphenadrine Citrate

➤ Chemically, it is N,N-Dimethyl-2-[(2-methylphenyl)-phenyl-methoxy]-ethanamine. It is a cholinergic antagonist. It is colourless, odourless, crystalline powder.

➤ Used in Parkinson's disease and as a skeletal muscle relaxant. It is an antihistaminic agent.

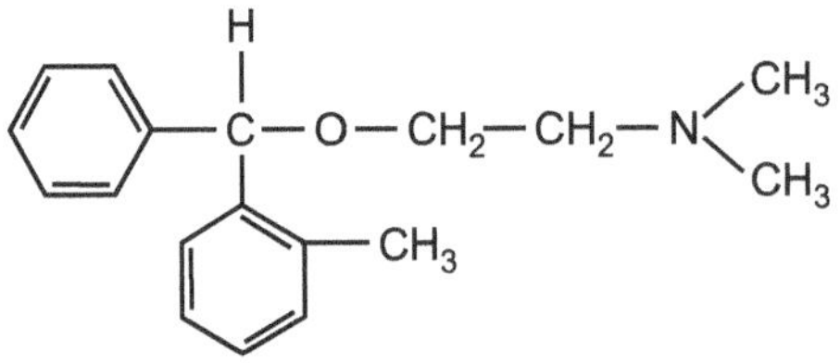

Orphenadrine citrate

3.12.10 Biperidine Hydrochloride

➤ Chemically, it is 1-(bicyclo[2.2.1]hept-5-en-2-yl)-1-phenyl-3-(piperidin- 1-yl)propan-1-ol.

➤ Used to treat Parkinson's disease, tremor and rigidity. It is an antipsychotic drug.

Biperidin hydrochloride

3.12.11 Procyclidine Hydrochloride

➢ Chemically, it is 1-cyclohexyl-1-phenyl-3-pyrrolidin-1-yl-propan-1-ol hydrochloride. It is a cholinergic antagonist and effective peripherially.

➢ Used in the treatment of Parkinson's disease.

Procyclidine hydrochloride

Synthesis:

It is synthesised from acetophenone, formaldehyde and pyrrolidine which is then treated with Grignard reagent to give procyclidine hydrochloride.

Acetophenone

Procyclidine hydrochloride

3.12.12 Tridihexethyl Chloride

➢ Chemically, it is 3-cyclohexyl-N,N,N-triethyl-3-hydroxy-3-phenylpropan-1-aminium. It is a muscarinic anticholinergic agent.

➢ Used in Parkinson's disease and ulcer. Also used as antispasmodic.

Tridihexethyl chloride

3.12.13 Isopropamide Iodide

➢ Chemically, it is 4-amino-N,N-diisopropyl-N-methyl-4-oxo-3,3-diphenylbutan-1-aminium.

➢ It is an anticholinergic, antispasmodic drug and having longer duration of action.

➢ Used to treat peptic ulcer, GI disorders.

Isopropamide iodide

3.12.14 Ethopropazine Hydrochloride

➢ Chemically, it is 10-[2-(Diethylamino)propyl]phenothiazine hydrochloride. It is an inhibitor of butyryl cholinesterases.

➢ Used in the treatment of Parkinson's disease.

Ethopropazine hydrochloride

QUESTIONS

1. What are cholinergic blocking agents? Give its classification. Explain the SAR of acetyl choline with examples.
2. Outline the synthesis of Dicyclomine.
3. What are cholinergic agents? Discuss cholinesterase inhibitors in detail.
4. Write a note on neuromuscular blocking agents with at least two structures.
5. Give an account of chemistry and biological activity of cholinergic agents.
6. Classify synthetic cholinergic blocking agents. Outline the synthesis of Dicyclomine.
7. Add a note on irreversible cholinestererase inhibitors.
8. What are parasympatholytic agents and how are they classified?
9. Write a brief note on indirectly acting cholinergic agonist.
10. Write a brief note on ganglionic blocking agents.
11. Give a brief account of muscarinic and nicotinic receptors.
12. Outline the synthesis of pyridostigmine.

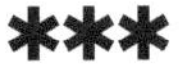

DRUGS ACTING ON CENTRAL NERVOUS SYSTEM

♦ LEARNING OBJECTIVES ♦

After completing this unit, reader should be able to understand:

❖ To study definition, classification and mechanism of action of hypnotic and sedative.

❖ To study benzodiazepine, its metabolism and structure-activity relationship in detail.

❖ To study various drugs of benzodiazepine derivatives with their uses.

❖ To learn barbiturates, its synthetic pathway, metabolism and structure-activity relationship.

❖ To study in brief about the miscellaneous class of hypnotics and sedative.

❖ To learn the synthetic scheme of some selected hypnotics and sedative.

❖ To know about epilepsy/convulsion with its types.

❖ To learn detail classification, mechanism of action and structure-activity relationship of anticonvulsant drugs.

(A) SEDATIVES AND HYPNOTICS

4.1 INTRODUCTION

In general sedative-hypnotics are drugs used to slow down mental and physical functions of the body. These are also referred to as CNS depressants. Sedatives are chemical agents tend to produce a calming effect, relax muscles, and relieve feelings of tension, anxiety, and irritability without causing drowsiness or sleep. Example: Potassium bromide.

At higher doses, most of these sedative drugs will also produce drowsiness and eventually produce sleep. Drugs that have such a sleep-inducing effect or producing sleep similar to that of natural sleep are called hypnotic drugs or hypnotics, commonly known as sleeping pills, are a class of psycho-depressive drugs. Example: Thiopentone sodium.

There is no sharp distinction between sedative and hypnotics and the same drug may have both actions depending on the method of use and the dose employed. At lower dose, the drug may act as sedative while at a higher dose the same drug may act as hypnotics. However, the combination of the terms sedative-hypnotic appropriately identifies the major pharmacological effects of these drugs. In reality, almost any drug that calms, soothes, and reduces anxiety is also capable of relieving insomnia and also frequently used in pre-anaesthetic medication and as an adjunctive therapy in psychiatry. Although the narcotics and sedative-hypnotics share many of the same actions, the latter drugs have no practical pain-relieving properties. Unlike the narcotics, intoxicating doses of the sedative-hypnotics almost always result in impaired judgement, slurred speech, and loss of motor function.

4.2 CLASSIFICATION OF SEDATIVES AND HYPNOTICS

1. **Benzodizepine derivatives:** Chlordiazepoxide, Diazepam, Oxazepam, Chlorazepate, Alprozolam, Lorazepam, Zolpidem.
2. **Barbiturates:** Barbital, Phenobarbital, Mephobarbital, Amobarbital, Butabarbital, Pentobarbital, Secobarbital.
3. **Miscellaneous:**
    (a) **Amides and imides:** Glutethimide.
    (b) **Aldehydes and their derivatives:** Paraldehyde, Triclofos sodium.
    (d) **Alcohols and their carbamate derivatives:** Ethchlorvynol, meprobamate.

4.3 BENZODIAZEPINES

Benzodiazepines have sedative, hypnotic, anti-anxiety, anticonvulsant, and muscle relaxant properties. Benzodiazepines have been used therapeutically since the early 1950s and were initially a part of a class of therapeutic agents referred to as tranquilizers. The "new" benzodiazepine agents were safer than the older barbiturate agents with far less addiction potential. Presently, benzodiazepines are referred to as sedative-hypnotic agents and have a number of different therapeutic uses including treatment of anxiety disorders, insomnia, seizure disorders, alcohol withdrawal symptoms and for conscious sedation or general anaesthesia. However, the use of BZDs is often controversial as they are widely acknowledged to be addictive and withdrawal symptoms can occur after 4-6 weeks of continuous use. This had led to the recommendation that they should not be used as hypnotics or anxiolytics for longer than 4 weeks.

They replaced barbiturates and meprobamate in the treatment of anxiety, because they are safer (less side effects and dependence) and more effective. At low doses they are useful as sedatives and at high doses they produce a hypnotic effect.

4.3.1 Classification of Benzodiazepines

Classification of benzodiazepines are classified according to duration of action into:

1. **Short acting (3-8 hours):** Triazolam, Oxazepam.
2. **Intermediate (10-20 hours):** Alprazolam, Lorazepam, Estazolam, Temazepam.

3. Long acting: (1-3 days): Diazepam, Chlordiazepoxide, Flurazepam, Quazepam, Clorazepate.

Chlordiazepoxide　　　　　**Diazepam**

Oxazepam　　　　**Lorazepam**　　　　**Zolpidem**

4.3.2 Mechanism of Action of Benzodiazepine

Mechanism of action: The great breakthrough in our understanding in the mechanism of action of BZDs came in the mid-1970s when biologists at Hoffman-La Roche demonstrated that BZDs exert their psychotropic effects by Gamma-Aminobutyric acid (GABA) is the major inhibitory neurotransmitter in the mammalian central nervous system (CNS), eliciting its physiological effects through interaction with several distinct classes of cell-surface receptors: $GABA_A$, $GABA_B$ and $GABA_C$ receptors. The $GABA_A$ receptor is the most abundant and is a member of the super family of ligand-gated ion channels. The interaction of GABA with this receptor determines the opening of the intrinsic chloride ion selective channel, which is followed by an increase in chloride flux, with the result of a hyperpolarization of the neuronal cell membrane and a concomitant decrease in neuronal transmission.

The $GABA_A$ receptor complex also has other distinct, high-affinity binding sites able to modulate the channel function, such as the benzodiazepine receptor (BzR), the picrotoxin site, the barbiturate site and sites that bind neurosteroids, and ethanol. All of these other sites are "allosteric" and function as modulatory sites that regulate GABA affinity. Among the allosteric receptor sites the sites for the benzodiazepines (BZD) are of prime importance since these ligands have been employed widely as anxiolytic/anticonvulsant agents since the 1960s. Studies of molecular biology have suggested that the $GABA_A$/BzR complex is a heteropentameric protein polymer constituted principally from α, β and γ subunits. At present, a total of 16 subunits (6α, 4β, 3γ, 1δ, and 2ρ) have been isolated and identified from the CNS (15 of these have been found in the mammalian CNS). Recent studies of recombinant $GABA_A$/BzR have shown that the presence of α, β and γ subunits is necessary to constitute a fully functional benzodiazepine receptor/GABA/chloride ion channel which mimics the pharmacological, biochemical, and electrophysiological properties of a native receptor.

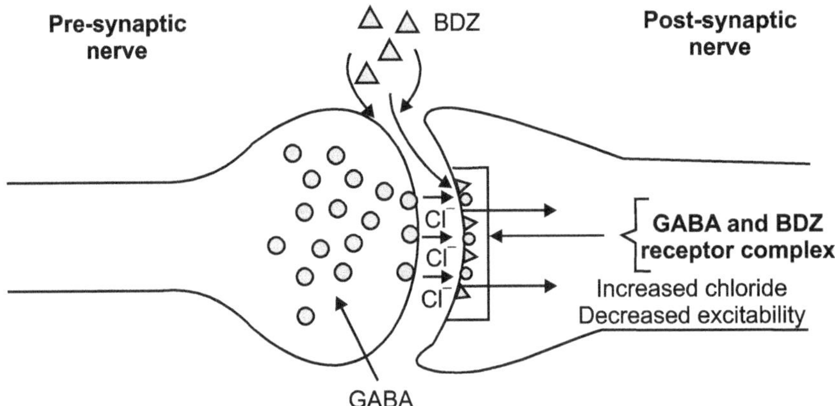

4.3.3 Structural Activity of Benzodiazepine

Benzodiazepines are the bicyclic heterocycles which contain a benzene nucleus being fused to a seven membered hetero ring having two nitrogen atoms, five carbon atoms and maximum possible number of cumulative double bonds. "Benzo" prefix benzene ring fused onto the diazepin ring. "R" labels denote common locations of side chains, which give different benzodiazepines with different properties.

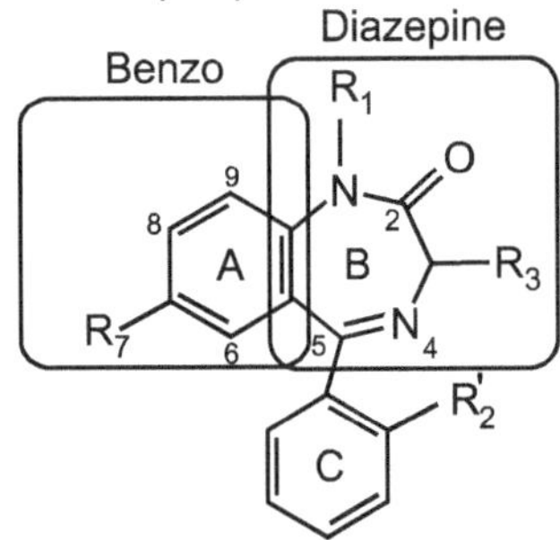

(1-Phenyl-1,4-benzodiazepin-2-one)

(1-phenyl-1,4-benzodiazepin-2-one)

Rings A, B and C are required for BDZ-receptor binding activity:

Ring A participates in "pi-pi stacking" interactions with a complimentary functionality on the receptor.

➢ An electron withdrawing group or electronegative group at R_7 (usually Cl, Br, NO_2, or CN) is required for optimal receptor affinity and enhances the activity.

$$NO_2 > Br > CF_3 > Cl$$

➢ Substitution on other positions (6,8 and 9) of this ring may decrease activity.

Ring C contributes to BDZ-receptor binding through hydrophobic and steric interactions:

➢ Position $R_{2'}$ may be unsubstituted or contain a halogen atoms. Halogenations (F, Cl) generally increase BDZ activity.

➢ Substitution on other positions of this ring may decrease activity (4').

Ring B is required for optimal BDZ-receptor binding,

➢ R_1 can be H, CH_3, or relatively small alkyl groups show optimal activity.

➢ Amide can be replaced with an amidine group as in chlordiazepoxide.

➢ Amide can be replaced with heterocycle such as imidazole or triazole results in pharmacologically active benzodiazepine derivative with highest affinity.

➢ A proton accepting group (carbonyl oxygen) at 2-position is necessary to interact with receptor histidine residue that act as proton donor and help in ligand binding. Electron donating group must be in the same plane with electronegative group on ring A, favouring a coplanar spatial orientation of two moieties Substitution of O with S effect selective binding GABA BZR sub-populations but anxiolytic activity is maintained.

➢ Neither the amide C=O nor N-alkyl groups (R_1) directly contribute to binding. If replacement of the carbonyl function with two hydrogens in position-2 gives medazepam, less effective than diazepam.

➢ Substitution of 3-position methylene or imine nitrogen is sterically unfavourable. Derivatives having 3-hydroxy moiety have comparable potency to non-hydroxylated analogue but are excreted faster.

➢ The 4-5-imino group is not required for activity.

➢ Saturation of the 4,5-double bond reduces potency, as does a shift of the unsaturation into the 3,4-position.

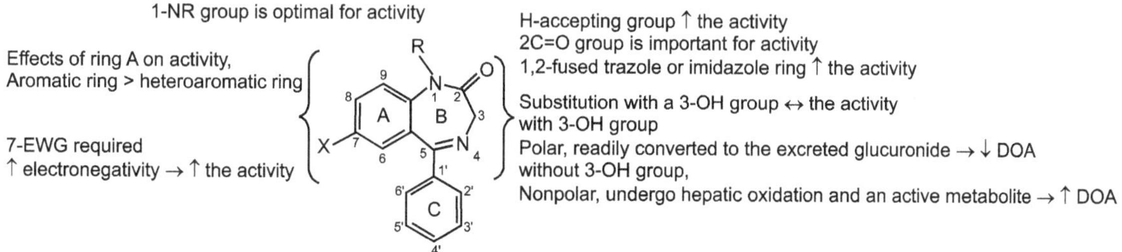

N-1-Substituted-3-Unsubstituted Benzodiazepines ("Diazepams")

Diazepam   **Prazepam**   **Flurazepam**

Halazepam   **Quazepam**   **Flunitrazepam**

Aminidino-N-oxide Benzodiazepines (Chlordiazepoxide)

Chlordiazepoxide

3-Carboxyl-N-1-Unsubstituted Benzodiazepines (Chlorazepate)

Chlorazepate

N-1-Substituted-3-Hydroxy Benzodiazepines ("N-Alkyl-Oxazepams")

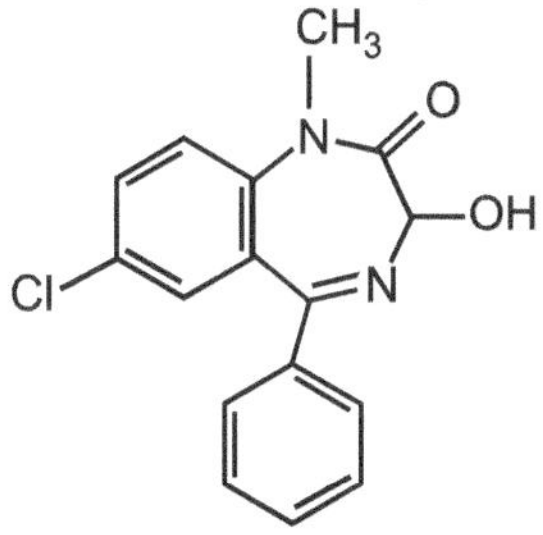

Temazepam

N-1-Unsubstituted-3-Hydroxy Benzodiazepines ("Oxazepams")

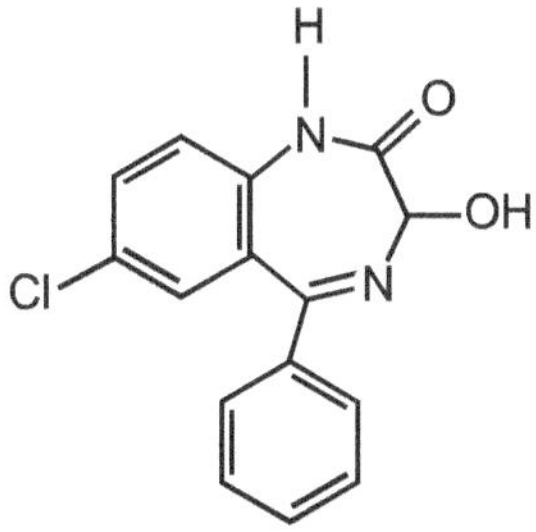

Oxazepam 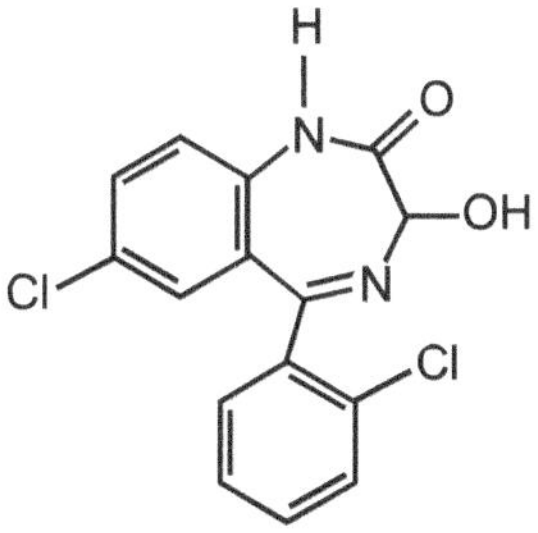   **Lorazepam**

Imidazo-Benzodiazepines

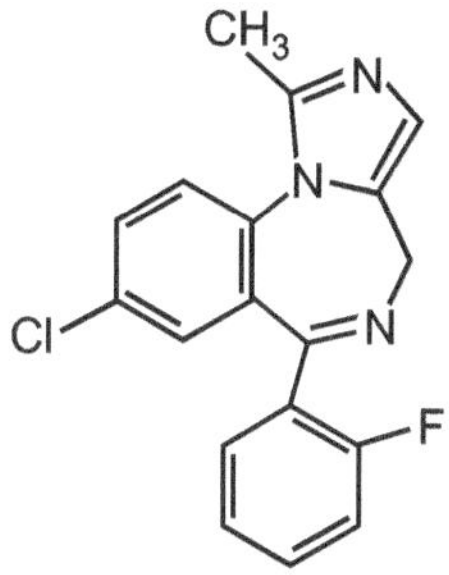

Midazolam

Triazolo-Benzodiazepines

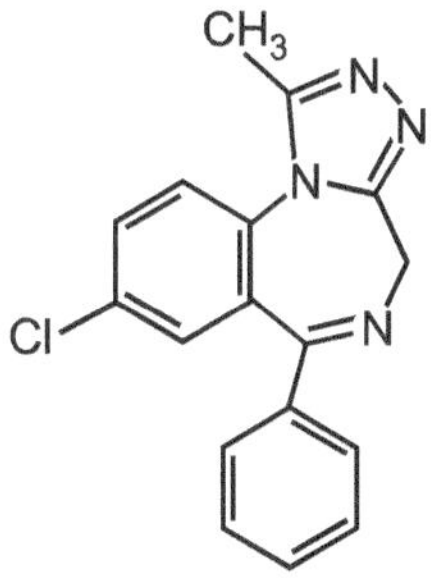

Alprazolam 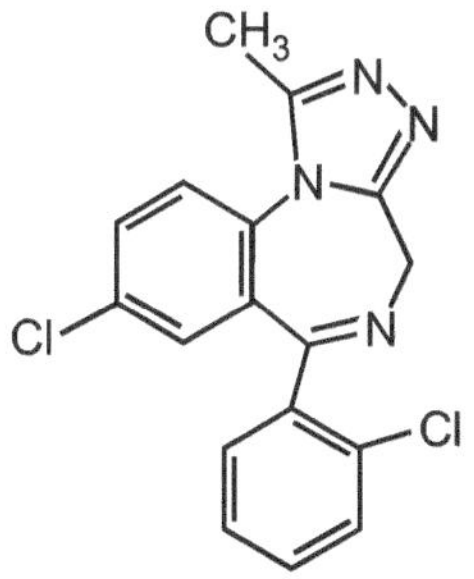   **Triazolam** 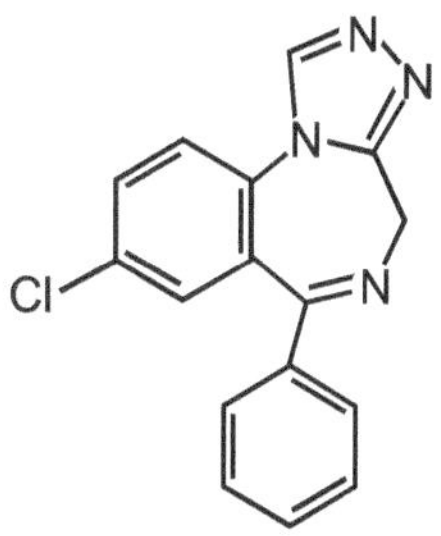   **Estazolam**

4.3.4 Clinical Uses of Benzodiazepines

➢ Anxiety disorders: Generalized anxiety disorder, acute anxiety, panic disorder, phobias (social, simple), post-traumatic stress disorder and obsessive-compulsive disorder.

- Anxiety associated with medical illness: Gastrointestinal, cardiovascular, and somatoform disorder.
- Insomnia.
- Convulsive disorders.
- Acute status epileptics: Neonatal seizures or febrile, tetanus, convulsions preeclampsia.
- Adjunct to other anticonvulsants.
- Amnestic (before surgery or procedure).
- Spastic disorders and other types of acute muscle spasms, multiple sclerosis, cerebral palsy, paraplegia secondary to spinal trauma.
- Involuntary movement disorders, restless leg syndrome, akathisia associated with neuroleptic use, myoclonus, choreform disorders.
- Detoxification from alcohol and other substances.
- Agitation or anxiety associated with other psychiatric conditions, psychotic illness, acute mania, anxiety associated with depression, impulse control disorders, catatonia or mutism.
- Diagnostic studies such as magnetic resonance imaging, computed tomography and endoscopic cardio version chemotherapy.

4.3.5 Basicity and Reactivity of Benzodiazepines

The BDZs are weak organic bases with the most basic nitrogen being the imine N_4 (amide at positions 1,2 is non-basic). Thus BDZ salts can only be formed with strong acids. Unfortunately, such strong acid salts are unstable and readily undergo sequential hydrolysis, first at the imine bond and then at the amide to yield inactive products. The first hydrolysis reaction (imine hydrolysis) is reversible; however the second (amide hydrolysis) eliminates GABA receptor activity.

4.3.6 Benzodiazepine Stereochemistry

Most BDZs do not have a chiral center, but the 7-membered B ring in these compounds may adopt one of two energetically preferred boat conformations (I and II below) which are enantiomeric relative to each other. Some studies suggest conformation I is preferred for BZD receptor binding:

Benzodiazepine Lipophilicity:

As a class the benzodiazepines are relatively lipophilic compounds due to their high hydrocarbon content and presence of halogen atoms. Also, most (not all) benzodiazepines do not behave as acids or bases under physiologic conditions and thus are not ionized.

Basicity and Reactivity of "Imidazo- and Triazolo-Benzodiazepines":

The tricyclic benzodiazepines have a more basic nitrogen atom (or more) in their additional ring structure (imidazole or triazole ring). These nitrogen atoms typically are not sufficiently basic to be protonated (ionized) at physiologic pH, but they are sufficiently basic to yield water soluble salts when treated with strong acids.

The salts formed from the heterocyclic benzodiazepines are more stable. When placed in aqueous media the heterocyclic salts may undergo imine hydrolysis similar to the traditional agents (see above), however no further hydrolysis (to inactive products) can occur since the heterocyclic compounds no longer have an acid labile amide group; in these compounds the amide was replaced with the heterocyclic group. Thus at acidic pH imine hydrolysis may occur as shown below but the reaction does not proceed, and at physiologic pH (post-injection) reformation of the benzodiazepine ring is favored as shown below:

Imidazo / Triazolo-BDZs   **Not hydrolyzed further**

Clorazepate and 3-Carboxylate Benzodiazepines: Prodrugs:

The 3-carboxylate benzodiazepines are unique in that they contain a 3-COO K^+ functionality which allows for water solubility. These drugs, of which chlorazepate is the prototype, function as water soluble prodrugs for the more traditional benzodiazepines. When administered (orally) they are readily protonated in the upper GI tract and spontaneously decarboxylate (loss of CO_2) as shown below to yield an active benzodiazepine which is absorbed from the gut. This is a chemical reaction and not an enzyme-catalyzed reaction

Chlorazepate   **Nordiazepam**

Flurazepam and 1-Alkylamino Benzodiazepines:

Flurazepam differs from other traditional benzodiazepines in that it contains a 1-(diethylamino)ethyl side chain. The nitrogen atom in this side chain is a typically tertiary amine and is relatively basic (pK_a about 9). Thus this nitrogen serves as a basic center for salt formation as shown below:

4.4 BENZODIAZEPINE PHARMACOKINETICS

Oral administration: Most BDZs are relatively weak bases and relatively lipophilic, resulting in fairly rapid and complete absorption from the GI tract. Absorption from other sites (IM) may be more erratic due to the lipophilicity of these compounds. Generally the rate of absorption from the GI tract is dependent on the lipophilicity of the BDZ. For example, diazepam is absorbed very rapidly, while oxazepam and clonazepam are absorbed more slowly.

Distribution: BDZs are highly protein bound (70-99%) but rapidly distribute to CNS. They cross the BBB by passive diffusion, thus the rate of CNS distribution correlates with lipophilicity (diazepam is "appropriately" lipophilic).

Duration of Action: The duration of BDZ action is dependent largely on the rate and nature of metabolism, which is dependent on the structure of the drug. Differences in duration are accounted for by structural differences involving primary N-1 and C-3-substitution and metabolism as detailed in the Metabolism Section. For example, compare diazepam and flurazepam (both N-substituted, non-C3-OH benzodiazepines) to oxazepam and lorazepam (N-unsubstituted, C3-OH benzodiazepines). It is also important to note that BDZs do not induce the metabolism of other drugs (unlike barbiturates).

BDZs and their metabolites may accumulate, especially upon repeated dosing. This may result in a delay in the appearance of adverse reactions, and extension the clinical effect beyond discontinuation of the drug. This creates concerns for hepatically impaired patients, elderly, etc.

4.4.1 Metabolism of Benzodiazepines

➤ **Metabolism of Chlordiazepoxide/Amidine BDZs: (Intermid Onset, Long Duration)**

Chlordiazepoxide is well absorbed after oral administration, but slowly and erratically absorbed from IM injection sites. This drug is metabolized to active benzodiazepine metabolites in a series of reactions beginning with CYP-mediated OND-demethylation of the amidine group. This "desmethyl" metabolite is slowly hydrolyzed to demoxepam which can undergo three different reactions:

(1) Hydrolysis to an inactive ring opened form

(2) Aromatic hydroxylation to phenol metabolites that retain some activity and

(3) Reduction to an active "nordiazepam" metabolite. The nordiazepam metabolite may be further oxidized to an active "oxazepam" metabolite that can be conjugated as a glucuronide which is inactive and eliminated.

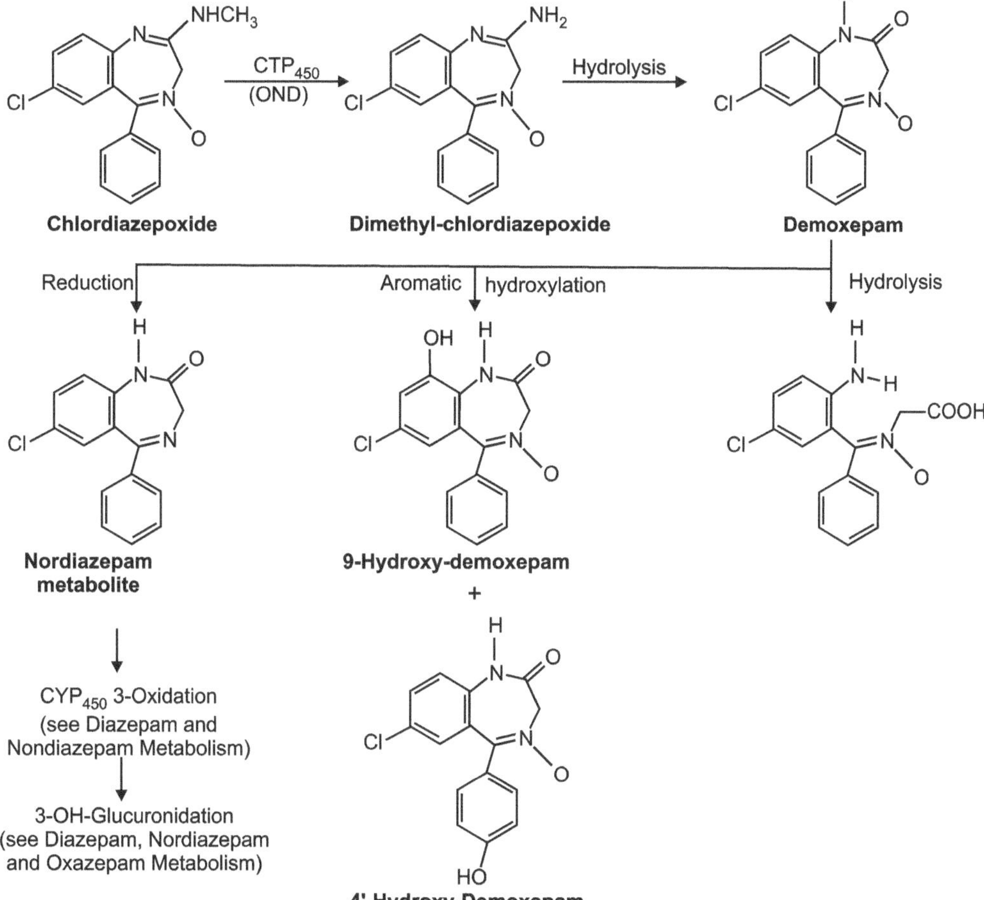

➤ **Metabolism of N-1-Substituted-3-Unsubstituted Benzodiazepines ("Diazepams"): Slow to fast onset and Long Duration**

The N-1-substituted-3-unsubstituted benzodiazepines or '"diazepams" are variably absorbed and distributed to the CNS based on their solubility and lipophilicity. All of these share the common property of long duration. This is a result of the formation of several active metabolites including the corresponding "nordiazepams" and "oxazepams" as shown in the figure. Each of these N-1-substituted-3-unsubstituted benzodiazepines undergo sequential oxidative metabolism, first at N-1 to yield active "nordiazepam" metabolites, then at the C-3 position to yield active "oxazepam" metabolites. Each of these metabolites can penetrate the BBB and enter the CNS and bind to BZ receptors on the GABA complex and thus are active. Each of these metabolites are also lipophilic enough to be reabsorbed from the kidney or during biliary cycling. Only after these benzodiazepines are metabolized to glucuronide conjugates is BZ-activity lost and the drug eliminated. Thus these compounds have long "effective" half-lives. It is important to note that the clearance of the N-1-substituted-3-unsubstituted benzodiazepines, as well as the amidine and 3-carboxyl benzodiazepines discussed above, is dependent on oxidative metabolism (largely hepatic metabolism). Thus elderly patients and others with impaired hepatic function will clear these drugs more slowly than benzodiazepines that do not require oxidation for clearance (see the "oxazepams" below). In other words, these benzodiazepines will have substantially longer half-lives and may accumulate in patients with impaired or limited hepatic function! It is also important to note that ONLY benzodiazepines with "oxidizable" N-1 substituent undergo N-1 oxidative dealkylation and that is why the carbon substituent bound to N-1 contains at least one (usually two) hydrogen atom. Benzodiazepine derivatives lacking hydrogen substitutents on the carbon bound to N-1 could not undergo this metabolic process.

➤ **Metabolism of 7-Nitro-benzodiazepines: Slow to intermediate onset and Long Duration**

As indicated in the metabolic scheme below, the 7-nitro-benzodiazepines can undergo the same metabolic reactions as other benzodiazepines of comparable functionality including OND at N-1 (when N-1 substituent is present), C-3-Oxidation and glucuronide conjugation of the C-OH metabolite. And again, the intermediate "nordiazepam" and "oxazepam" metabolites are active as BZ-receptor ligands, and these compounds thus have relatively long duration of action. The 7-nitro benzodiazepines also can undergo reduction of the 7-nitro group to the corresponding aniline (7-amino) as shown in the figure below. The 7-amino metabolites are typically less active than the parent nitro compounds (see structure-activity requirement), and can be conjugated by acetylation (also less active). Thus complex, inactive metabolites eventually form from these compounds:

- ➤ **Metabolism of Tricyclic Benzodiazepines: Relatively rapid onset, Intermediate to short duration**

These compounds are relatively lipophilic and thus are rapidly absorbed and diffused into the CNS. Metabolism of tricyclic benzodiazepines typically follows a different pathway than the "traditional" benzodiazepines. All of these compounds **except estazolam** have a "benzylic type" methyl group at the 1-position of the imidazole or triazole ring and this group is subject to rapid cytochrome-mediated oxidation as shown below. This 1-hydromethyl metabolite retains activity, but in most cases (**except alprazolam**) is rapidly conjugated as an inactive glucuronide and eliminated. Thus these compounds have intermediate to short duration of action. These compounds may also be oxidized at the available carbon in the benzodiazepine ring (as shown below), but this pathway appears to be relatively minor. Also some levels of the "ring-opened" benzophenone may exist in plasma (and appear in urine).

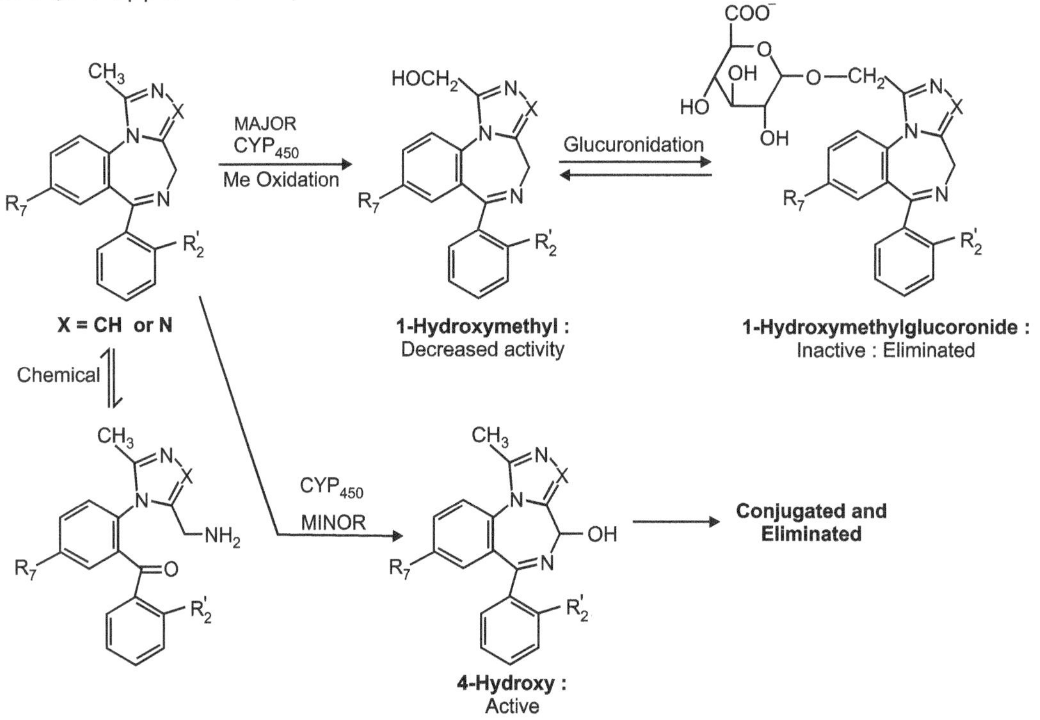

4.4.2 Benzodiazepine Derivatives

Chlordiazepoxide 7-chloro-2-(methylamino)-5-phenyl-3H-1,4-benzodiazepine 4-oxide hydrochloride.

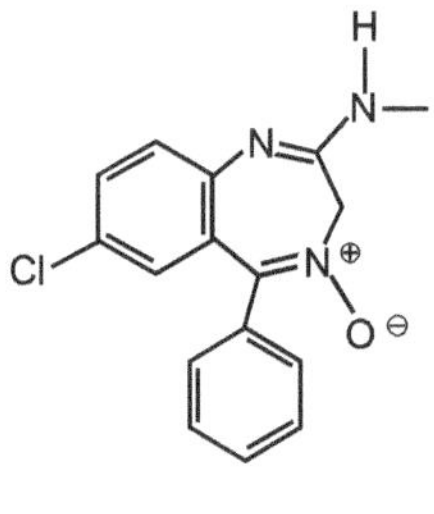

Chlordiazepoxide is a sedative and hypnotic drug belonging to benzodiazepine class. The half-life of the drug has a medium to long half life but its metabolite has a very long half-life.

Properties: The drug has amnesic, anticonvulsant, anxiolytic, hypnotic, sedative and skeletal muscle relaxant properties.

MOA: Allosteric $GABA_A$ enhancer.

Uses: It is used to treat anxiety, insomnia and withdrawal symptoms from alcohol and/or drug abuse.

Diazepam 7-chloro-1,3-dihydro-1-methyl-5-phenyl-1,4-benzodiazepine-2-one.

Diazepam

Long acting benzodiazepine (>20 hrs), due to high blood protein binding of 98.5% which reduces rate of elimination and its metabolic product is also active.

Properties: It has anxiolytic, anticonvulsant, hypnotic - sedative, skeletal muscle relaxant, and amnestic properties.

Uses: It is used as anxiety, panic attacks, insomnia, seizures, muscle spasms (such as in tetanus cases), restless legs syndrome, alcohol withdrawal, opiate withdrawal syndrome. It is also used as a premedication for inducing sedation, anxiolysis, or amnesia before certain medical procedures (e.g., endoscopy). Diazepam is the drug of choice for treating benzodiazepine dependence with its long half-life allowing easier dose reduction.

Not used for long term epilepsy due to development of tolerance and avoid during pregnancy.

MOA: Allosteric $GABA_A$ enhancer.

Synthesis: Friedel-Crafts acylation of 4-chloro aniline with corresponding benzoyl chloride in the presence of Lewis acid affects benzophenone derivative. Acetylation of an amino group with chloroacetyl chloride gives the chloro acetamide. Heating with ammonia undergoes cyclization reaction to form non-diazepam; N-methylation methyl iodide affords diazepam.

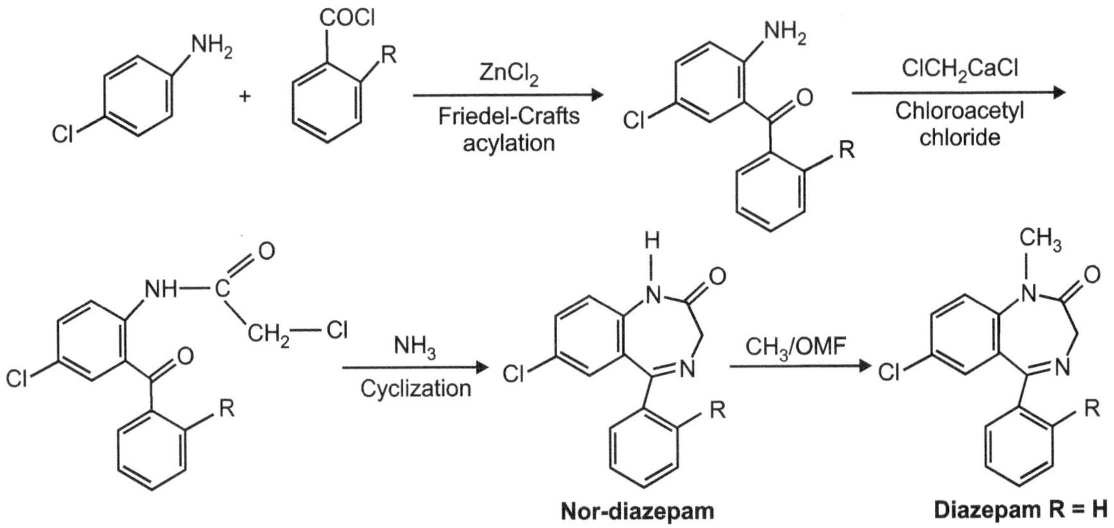

ZnCl$_2$ / Friedel-Crafts acylation

ClCH$_2$CaCl / Chloroacetyl chloride

NH$_3$ / Cyclization

CH$_3$/OMF

Nor-diazepam

Diazepam R = H

Oxazepam:

Oxazepam is a short acting benzodiazepine.

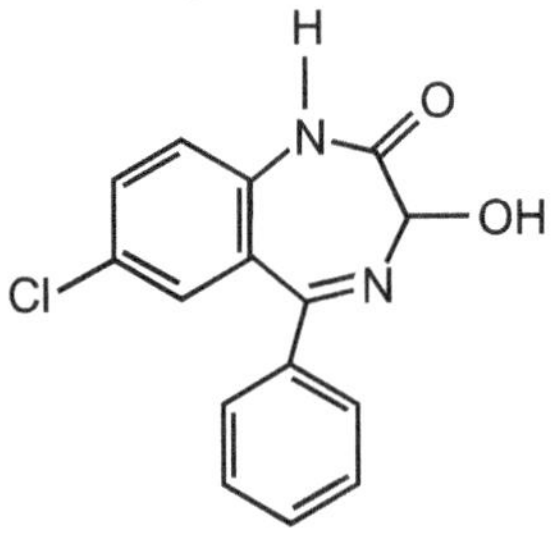

Properties: It is a metabolite of diazepam, prazepam and temazepam and has moderate amnesic, anxiolytic, anticonvulsant, hypnotic, sedative and skeletal muscle relaxant properties compared to other benzodiazepines.

Uses: It is used for the treatment of anxiety, insomnia and in the control of symptoms of alcohol withdrawal syndrome.

MOA: Allosteric GABA$_A$ enhancer.

Chlorazepate:

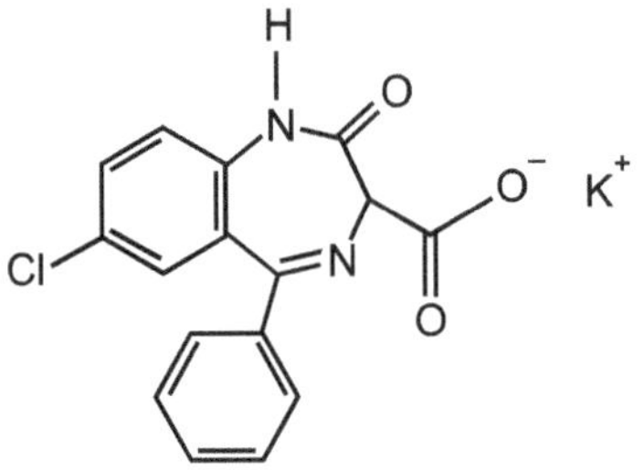

Chlorazepate is a benzodiazepine derivative. It is available as chlorazepate dipotassium.

Uses: Chlorazepate is used for symptomatic relief of anxiety associated with neurosis, phsychoneurosis.

MOA: Allosteric GABA$_A$ enhancer.

Lorazepam chemically, (E)-7-chloro-5-(2-chlorophenyl)-3-hydroxy-1H-benzo[1,4] diazepin-2(3H)-one.

Uses: It is used to treat anxiety disorders, trouble sleeping, active seizures including status epilepticus, alcohol withdrawal, and chemotherapy induced nausea and vomiting. It can be given by IV and the effect is showed between one and thirty minutes which last for upto a day.

Alprazolam 8-chloro-1-methyl-6-phenyl-4H-s-triazolo [4,3-a] [1,4] benzodiazepine.

Alprazolam is a triazolo analogue of 1,4-benzodiazepine. It belongs to intermediate acting benzodiazepine.

Properties: It has potent anxiolytic, amnestic, hypnotic, anticonvulsant, skeletal muscle relaxant, and sedative properties.

Uses: Alprazolam is used for the treatment of anxiety disorders and panic attacks can cause fetal abnormalities and should not be used in pregnancy. It is excreted in breast milk and should not be used by women who are nursing.

MOA: Alloteric $GABA_A$ enhancer.

4.4.3 Other Non-Benzodiazepine Sedatives

Zolpidem:

The zolpidem is not a benzodiazepine in structure, but it acts on a subset of the benzodiazepine receptor family.

Lorazepam, oxazepam and alprazolam have low hepatic metabolism and do not have active metabolites. Diazepam and chlorazepate are rapidly absorbed benzodiazepine agents and have the most rapid onset of action but also the greatest abuse/dependence potential. Chlordiazepoxide, clonazepam, clorazepate and diazepam are considered long-acting benzodiazepine agents and are associated with accumulation which may result in sedation, cognitive impairment and psychomotor retardation. Alprazolam and lorazepam are considered short-acting benzodiazepine agents and have been associated with increased anxiety, insomnia and rebound effects upon discontinuation. All benzodiazepine agents result in dependence or tolerance with long-term use. Benzodiazepine therapy should be discontinued by a slow taper to avoid withdrawal effects including: "sleep disturbance, irritability, increased tension and anxiety, panic attacks, hand tremor, sweating, difficulty in concentration, dry wretching and nausea, some weight loss, palpitations, headache, muscular pain" and may also include more serious effects including seizures and psychotic reactions. Transitioning patients from long-acting to short-acting agents may allow for more flexibility and aid in discontinuing therapy.

4.5 BARBITURATE

Barbiturates are a group of drugs in the class known as sedative-hypnotics. Barbiturates were first introduced in 1903 and became increasingly popular in the 1960s and 1970s as treatments for anxiety, insomnia, or seizure disorders. The abuse of barbiturates increased in a similar fashion. Barbiturate use and abuse has declined dramatically since the 1970s, primarily due to the advent of the safer benzodiazepines.

Barbiturates all have a similar structure (barbituric acid), but differing side chains influence the drug's potency, duration of effect, and rapidity of symptom onset.

4.5.1 Barbiturate General Structure and Numbering

Barbiturates contain a "balance" of hydrophilic (2,4,6-pyrimidinetrione ring structure) and lipophilic (5,5′-substituents) functionality. The overall hydrophilic (polar) or lipophilic (non-polar) character of the barbiturates is a function of:

- The hydrophilicity of the pyrimidinetrione ring which is a function of the number of N-substituents and the pK_a of the acidic proton(s), and
- The overall size and structure of the two substituents at the 5-position.

4.5.2 Classification of Barbiturates

Long-Acting Barbiturates:

Relatively slow onset (30-60 minutes) and relatively long duration (10-16 hours).

Structure: N-H or N-Methyl and C-5 side chains consisting of two ethyl groups, or an ethyl and phenyl group.

Properties: Relatively low lipophilicity and low plasma protein binding (<40%):

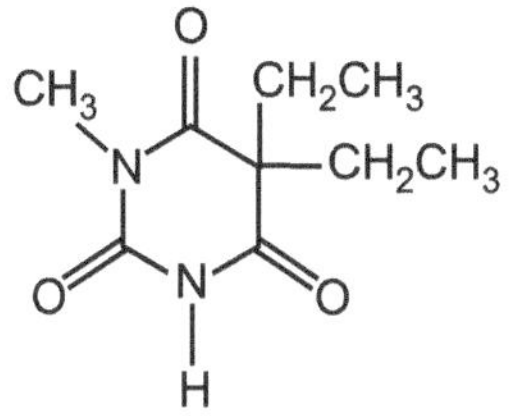

Metharbital 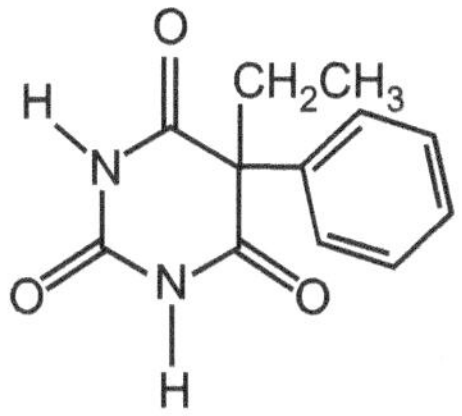   **Phenobarbital** 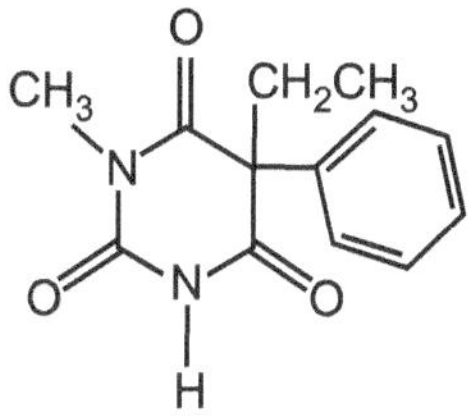   **Mephobarbital**

Intermediate-Acting Barbiturates:

Relatively slow onset (45-60 minutes) and intermediate duration (6-8 hours).

Structure: N-H and C-5 side substituents consisting of ethyl or allyl group and a 3 to 5-carbon atom unit.

Properties: Intermediate lipophilicity and intermediate plasma protein binding (50%).

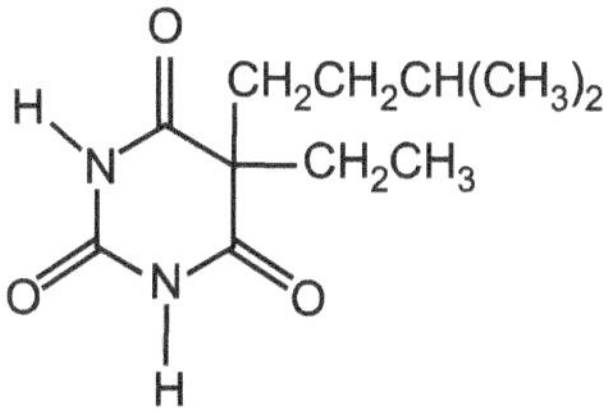

Amobarbital 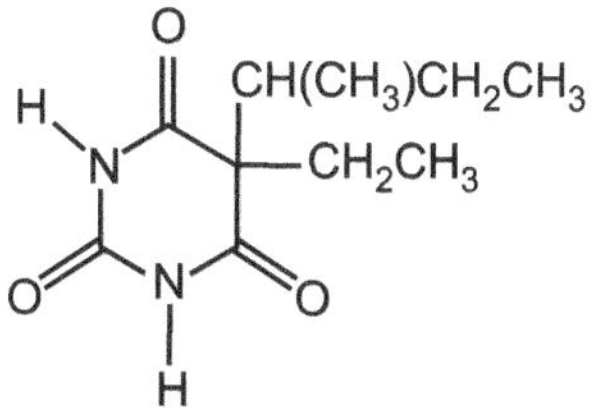   **Butabarbital**

Short-Acting Barbiturates:

Relatively rapid onset (10-15 minutes) and relatively short duration (3-4 hours).

Structure: N-H and C-5 side chains consisting of ethyl or allyl and a 5 carbon unit.

Properties: High lipophilicity and high plasma protein binding (70%). Rapid distribution and redistribution.

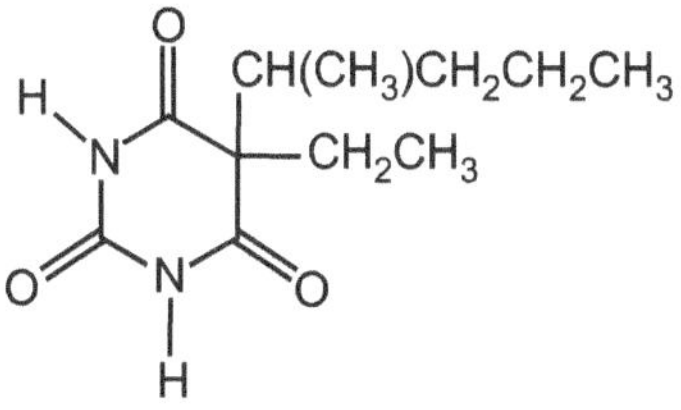

Pentobarbital
(Ethyl substituted)   **Secobarbital**
(Allyl substituted)

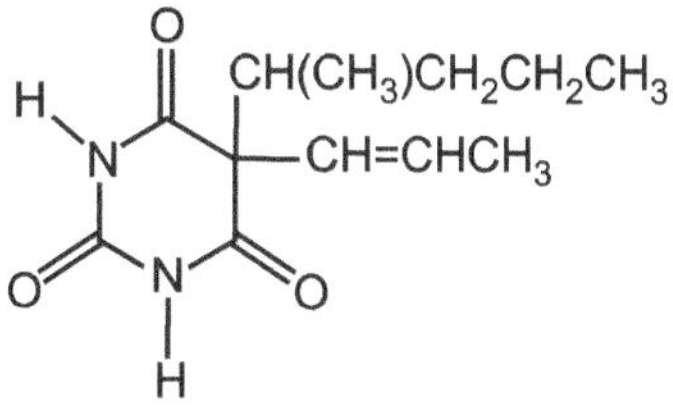

Ultra-Short-Acting Barbiturates:

Administered by injection (as salts): Immediate onset and very short duration.

Structure: N-H with a thiocarbonyl and C-5 side chains consisting of ethyl or allyl with a 5 carbon unit.

Properties: Very high lipophilicity and high plasma protein binding (>70%). Rapid distribution and redistribution.

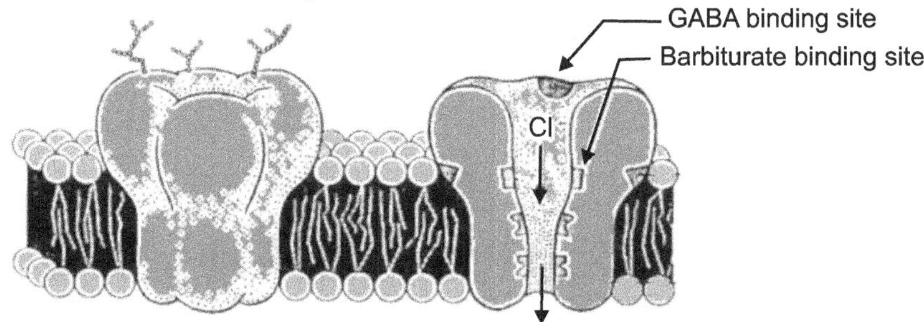

Thiopental
(Ethyl substituted)

Thiamylal
(Allyl substituted)

4.5.3 Barbiturates and Mechanism of Action

Barbiturates potentiate the effect of GABA at the GABA-A receptor. The GABA-A receptor is a ligand gated ion channel membrane receptor that allows for the flow of Cl^- through the membrane in neurons. GABA is the principle neurotransmitter for this receptor which upon binding causes the channel to open and create a negative change in the transmembrane potential. This makes it an inhibitory neurotransmitter.

Barbiturates also block the AMPA receptor which is sensitive to glutamate, the excitatory neurotransmitter. Glutamate performs the opposite effect from GABA restricting ion flow and increasing the transmembrane action potential of the neuron. By blocking this action, barbiturates serve to increase the duration of the receptor response to GABA and extend the depressed condition of the cell.

4.5.4 Structure-Activity Relationship of Barbiturates (SAR)

Barbiturate

One of the ways of making potentially biologically active compounds is modification on C-5 of barbituric acid. Combination of barbituric acid moiety with other pharmacophoric groups gives possibility to synthesize numerous derivatives with potential biological effect.

- Two active hydrogen atoms at position 5:5 have appropriate substituent (alkyl or aryl) group to produce hypnotic activity.

- The total number of carbon atoms present in the two groups at carbon 5 must not be less than 4 and more than 10 for the optimal therapeutic results.

- Only one of the substituent groups at position C-5 may be a closed chain. Methylepentobarbital.

- The branched chain isomer exhibits greater activity and shorter duration. The greater the branching, the more potent is the drug e.g., pentobarbital > amobarbital.

- Double bonds in the alkyl substituent groups produce compounds more readily vulnerable to tissue oxidation; hence, they are short-acting. e.g. Pentobarbital sodium.

- Aromatic and alicyclic moieties exert greater potency than the corresponding aliphatic moiety having the same number of carbon atoms. Methylepentobarbital

- Short chains at C-5 resist oxidation and hence are long-acting. Long chains are readily oxidized and thus produce short-acting barbiturates. Pentobarbital Sodium Barbital

- Inclusion of a halogen atom in the C-5 alkyl moiety enhances activity.

- Inclusion of polar groups (e.g., OH, CO, COOH, NH_2, RNH, and SO_3H) in the C-5 alkyl moiety reduces potency considerably.

- Methylation of one of the imide hydrogens enhances onset and reduces duration of action.

- The replacement of O-atom with an S-atom, at C-2 position of the barbiturates significantly enhances the lipid solubility profile. The resulting modified versions of the barbiturates thus obtained exert a rapid onset of activity by virtue of the fact that they attain maximal thiobarbiturate -brain levels. Therefore, such drugs as 'thiopental sodium' find their profuse and abundant application as 'intravenous anaesthetics'. Thiopental sodium.

- Inclusion of more sulphur atoms (e.g., 2, 4-dithio; 2, 4, 6-trithio) decreases activity. Likewise introduction of imino group(s) into the barbituric acids abolishes activity (e.g., 2-imino ; 4-imino ; 2, 4-diimino and 2, 4, 6-triimino).

4.5.5 Clinical Uses of Barbiturates

Sedation: Although traditionally used as non-specific CNS depressants for daytime sedation, the barbiturates have generally been replaced by the benzodiazepines.

Hypnotic: Short-term treatment of insomnia, since barbiturates appear to lose their effectiveness in sleep induction and maintenance after 2 weeks. If insomnia persists, seek alternative therapy (including non-drug) for chronic insomnia.

Anticonvulsant (mephobarbital, phenobarbital): Treatment of partial and generalized tonic-clonic and cortical focal seizures.

4.5.6 Barbiturate Ionization, Acidity and Salt Formation

Barbiturates containing at least one N-H hydrogen atom are acidic. Acidity results from the ability of the N to lose hydrogen and the stabilization of the resulting anionic charge of the conjugate base by resonance delocalization as shown below:

Acid form

Conjugate Base Resonance Forms

The relative acidity of different barbiturates is a function of the degree of N substitution and C-5-substitution as shown below (electron donors decrease acidity).

Barbituric acid : pK_a 4.12

5,5'-Disubstituted barbituric acid: pK_a 6.5-8

3,5,5'-Trisubstituted barbituric acid: pK_a > 8

- Barbituric acid (N- and C-5-unsubstituted) is the highly acidic (but not active as a CNS depressant): See structures above.

- Addition of substituents at the 5-position decrease acidity (raise pKa) due to the electron donating effects (+I) of the 5-alkyl groups: See structures above.

- Substitution at one ring nitrogen atom reduces acidity (raise pKa) due to the electron donating effects (+I) of the N-alkyl group: See structures above.

- Substitution at BOTH ring nitrogen atoms eliminates both acidic protons (non-acidic).

Due to the presence of one (or more) acidic protons, barbiturates can be converted to water soluble salt forms by treatment with an appropriate base as shown below. Note that the charge resides primarily on the more electronegative oxygen atom:

Acid form
Water insoluble

Salt form (conjugate base)
Water soluble

4.5.7 Barbiturate Chirality and Stereochemistry

The barbiturate ring system contains only one sp^2 carbon atom and it is not chiral unless (1) there are two different C-5 substituents and (2) one ring nitrogen is substituted as shown in the example below:

Achiral
(No chiral center)

Achiral
(No chiral center)

Achiral
(No chiral center)

Chiral C-5 carbon
(R&S enantiomers)

The C-5 substituents may contain chiral (unsymmetrically substituted sp^2 carbon atom(s)) and in such cases the barbiturate is chiral. Some barbiturates have both a chiral C-5 atom and a chiral side chain as shown in one example below.

Achiral
(No chiral center)

Chiral C-5 substituent
(R & S enantiomers)

Chiral C-5 carbon and
chiral C-5 substituent
(4 enantiomers possible)

4.5.8 Metabolism of Barbiturates

Barbiturates are distributed throughout the body with highest concentrations occurring in the brain, liver and kidneys. In general, duration of action is dependent upon lipid solubility and extent of protein binding with the short acting barbiturates showing the most lipid solubility and percentage of protein binding. The short and intermediate acting barbiturates are nearly entirely metabolized by the liver and excreted in the urine, while 25-50% of a dose of a long acting barbiturate is excreted as unchanged drug. The half-life is variable with short acting barbiturates being detectable in urine for 24 hours and the long acting drugs detectable for 2-3 weeks following ingestion.

A. Omega and Omega-1 Oxidation:

Enantiomeric alcohols possible

Examples : Most barbiturates

C. Alkene and Allylic Oxidation:

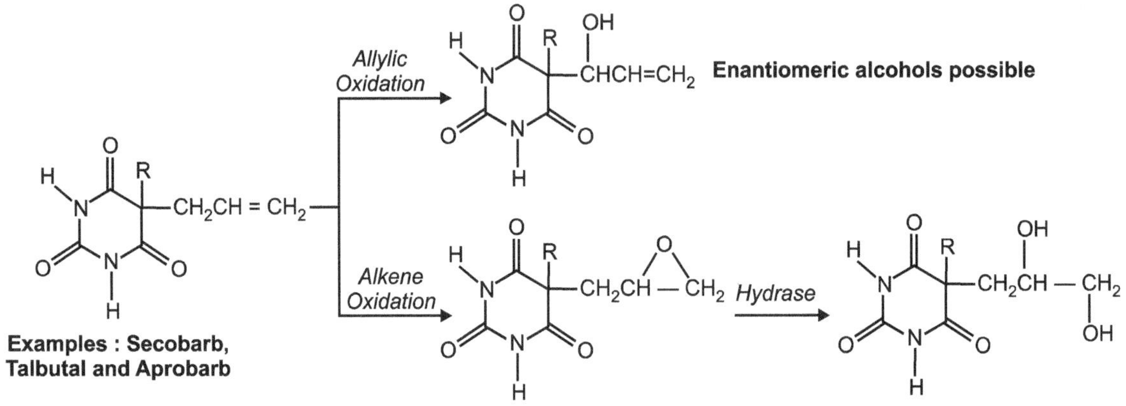

**Examples : Secobarb,
Talbutal and Aprobarb**

Examples: Secobarb, Talbutala nd aprobarb.

D. N-oxidation:

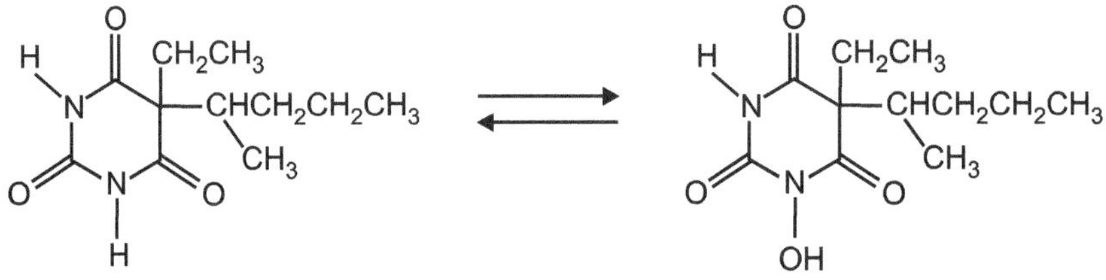

Most Barbs

E. Desulfuration:

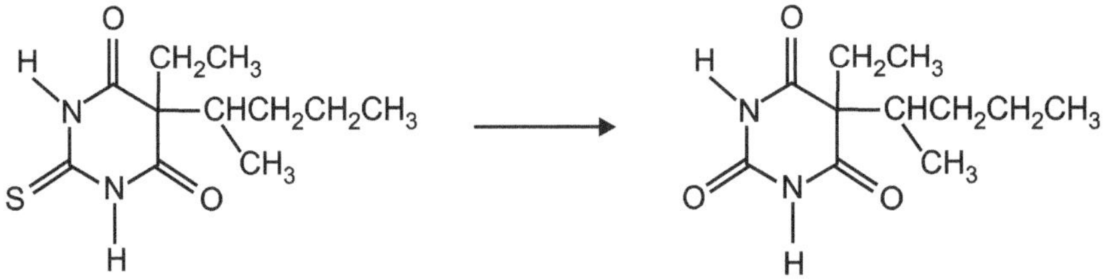

Thiobarbs

F. Oxidation N-dealkylation:

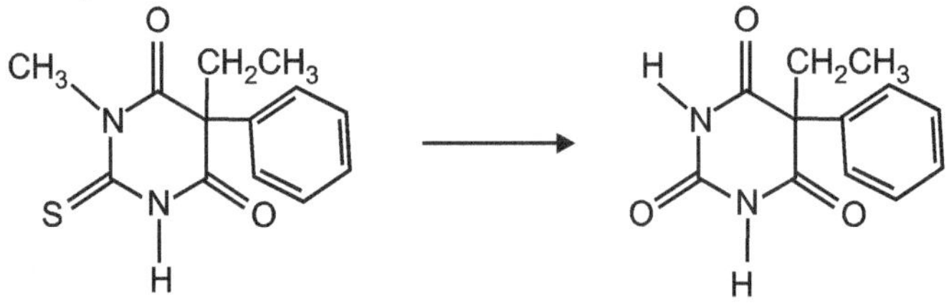

N-methylbarbs

G. Hydrolysis:

Most Barbs

4.5.9 Barbiturate Derivatives

Barbital

Chemistry: Barbital is 5,5-diethylbarbituric acid.

Properties: Barbital is a white crystalline powder. It is slightly soluble in water but freely soluble in aqueous solutions of alkali hydroxides and carbonates. It is prepared by condensation of ethyl diethylmalonate with urea.

Phenobarbitone/Phenobarbital, 5-ethyl-5-phenylbarbituric acid. It occurs as sodium salt.

Properties: Phenobarbitone sodium is hygroscopic, bitter taste, water soluble, odourless, white crystalline powder.

Synthesis: Phenobarbitone is synthesized by the following steps:

- In the first step a β-keto ester (Ethyl oxalophenylacetate) is prepared by Claisen condensation reaction of ethylphenylacetate with ethyloxalate in presence of sodium.

- The ethyl oxalophenylacetate is then decomposed by distillation to form ethylphenylmalonate. The ethyl phenylmalonate is further ethylated to form ethyl ethylphenylmalonate with ethyl bromide and ethanol.

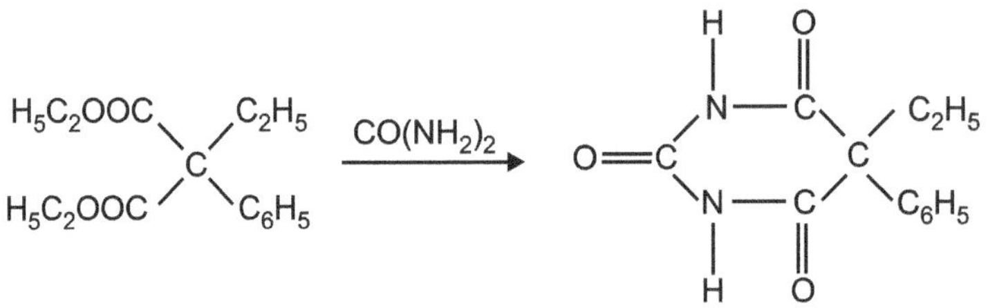

Phenobarbitone

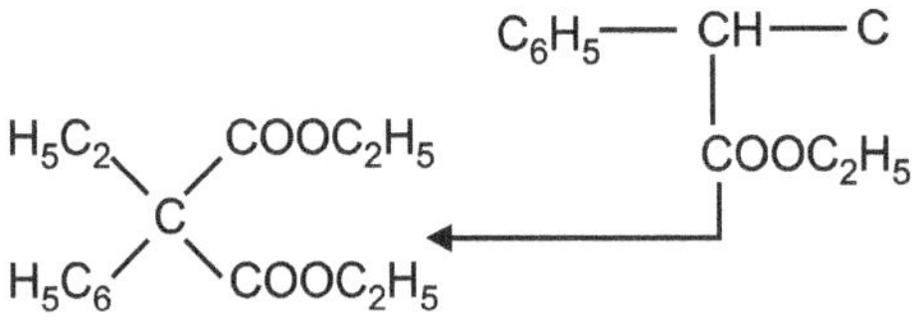

Methyl Phenobarbitone (Mephobarbital):

Chemistry: Methyl phenobarbitone is 5-ethyl-1-methyl-5-phenylbarbituric acid synthesis.

Mephobarbital is prepared by condensing ethylphenyl ethyl malonate with monomethyl urea.

Properties: Mephobarbital is a white crystalline, water insoluble powder. It is soluble in aqueous solutions of alkali hydroxides and carbonates.

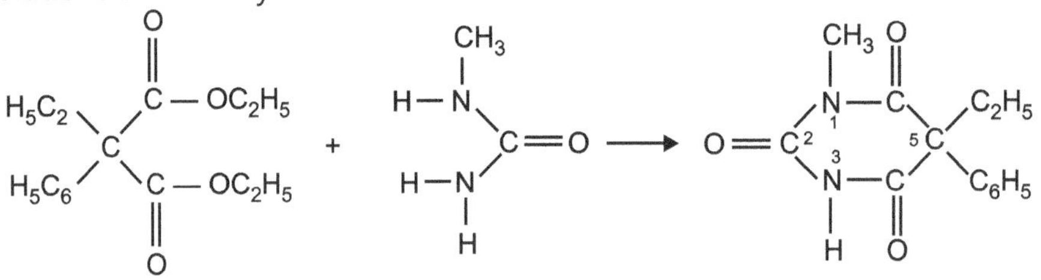

Methylphenobarbitone

Amobarbitone / Amobarbital:

Chemistry: Amobarbitone is 5-ethyl-5-isopentylbarbituric acid.

Properties: It occurs as a white crystalline powder. It is slightly soluble in water but freely soluble in alkali hydroxide and carbonate solutions. It is prepared by condensation of ethyl isopentyl ethylmalonate with urea.

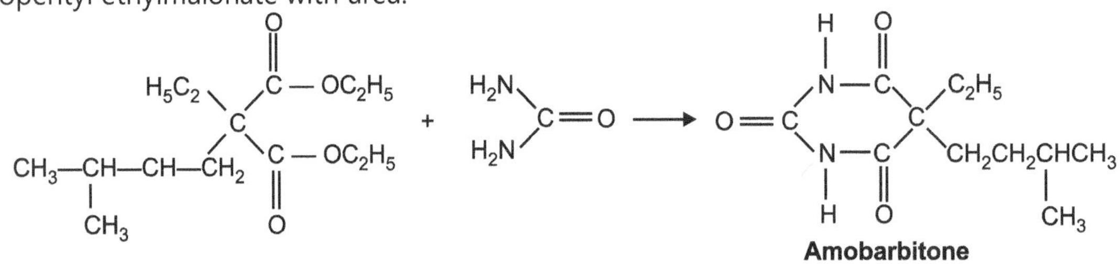

Amobarbitone

Butobarbitone / Butobarbital:

Chemistry: Butobarbitone is 5-isobutyl-5-ethylbarbituric acid.

Properties: It is white crystalline powder, slightly soluble in water. It is prepared by condensation of ethyl isobutyl ethylmalonate with urea.

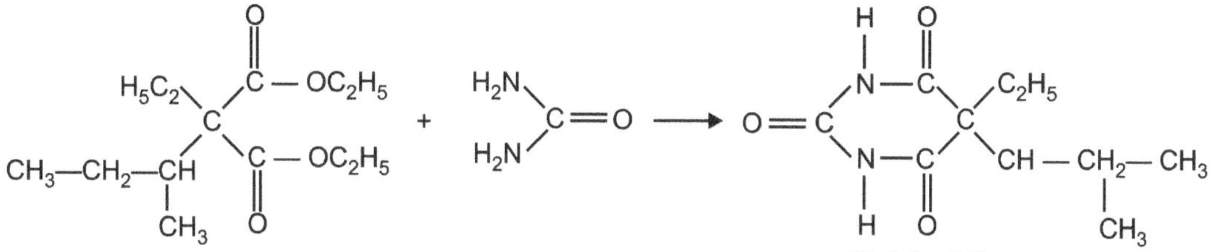

Butobarbitone

Pentobarbitone / Pentobarbital:

Chemistry: Pentobarbitone is 5-ethyl-5-(1-methylbutyl) barbituric acid. Pento-barbitone is available as pentobarbitone sodium salt. It is prepared by condensing ethyl 1-metyl butylethyl malonate with urea.

Properties: Pentobarbitone and its sodium salt is available as white, crystalline powder. Pentobarbitone is slightly soluble in water, whereas its sodium salt is freely soluble in water.

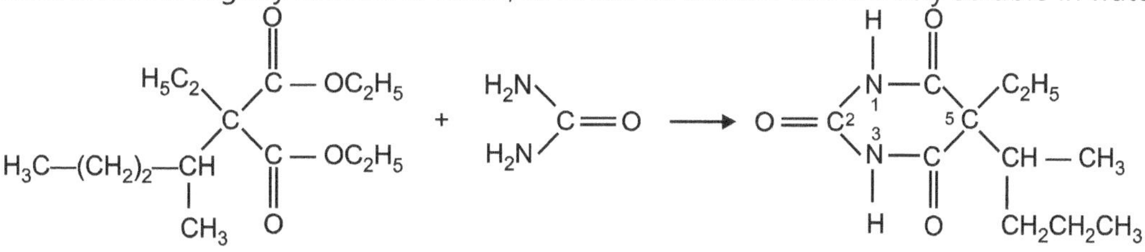

Pentobarbitone

Secobarbitone / Secobarbital:

Chemistry: It is also known as Quinalbarbitone. Quinalbarbitone is (RS)-5-allyl-5-(1-methylbutyl) barbituric acid. It is prepared by condensing equimolar mixture of urea with ethyl 1-methylbutylmalonate and alkyl bromide.

Properties: Quinalbarbitone occurs as its sodium salt. Quinalbarbitone sodium is a white powder. It is freely soluble in water.

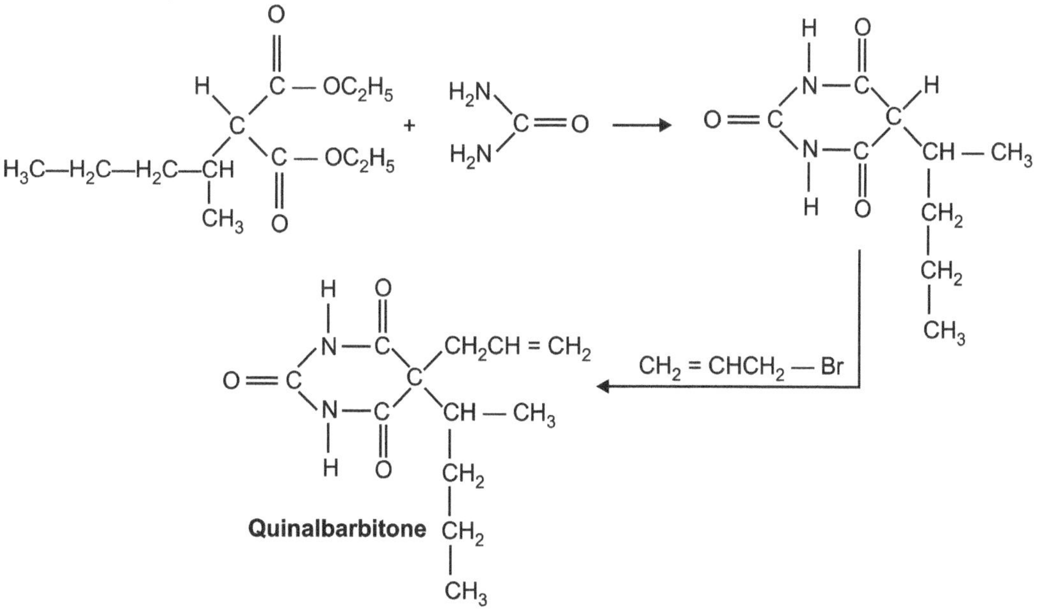

Quinalbarbitone

4.6 NON-BARBITURATE

Numerous heterocyclic derivatives with low toxicity for hypnotic and sedative properties were synthesized. The following are some most important non-barbiturate sedative-hypnotics among piperidines, quinazolinones, aldehydes, benzodiazepines etc.

4.6.1 Amides and Imides

Glutethimide 2-ethyl-2-phenyl-glutarimide.

Barbiturate

Glutethimide
(Piperidine - 2, 6-dione)

Structure, Chemistry and Actions: A barbiturate analogue lacking one of the "amide components" of the typical barbiturate ring system. Glutethimide is similar to the barbiturates including the presence of an acidic imide group (pKa 9.2). It produces CNS depression similar to the barbiturates. Glutethimide exhibits pronounced anticholinergic activity, which is manifested by mydriasis, inhibition of salivary secretions and decreased intestinal motility. It has generally been replaced by safer and more effective agents.

Glutethimide is prepared by the following steps:

Step 1: Glutethimide is prepared by treating benzyl cyanide with ethyl chloride in presence of sodamide to yield α-ethyl benzyl cyanide.

Step 2: The above formed α-ethyl benzyl cyanide is condensed with α-bromopropionic ester to form substituted hexanoic acid.

Substituted hexanoic acid

Step 3: Cyclization. Substituted hexanoic acid forms the amide on treatment with 80% H_2SO_4 which spontaneously cyclizes to glutethimide.

Substituted hexanoic acid

Glutethimide

Properties: Gultethemide is colorless or white colored, water insoluble powder. It should be stored in light protected containers.

Uses: Gultethimide is used as hypnotic in all types of insomnia. It induces sleep without depressing respiration.

Absorption/Distribution: It is erraticallly absorbed from the GI tract giving peak plasma concentration within 1-6 hours after administration. The average plasma half-life is 10 to 12 hours. About 50% of the drug is bound to plasma proteins; protein binding results in part from modest acidity (imide) Glutethimide stimulates hepatic microsomal enzymes.

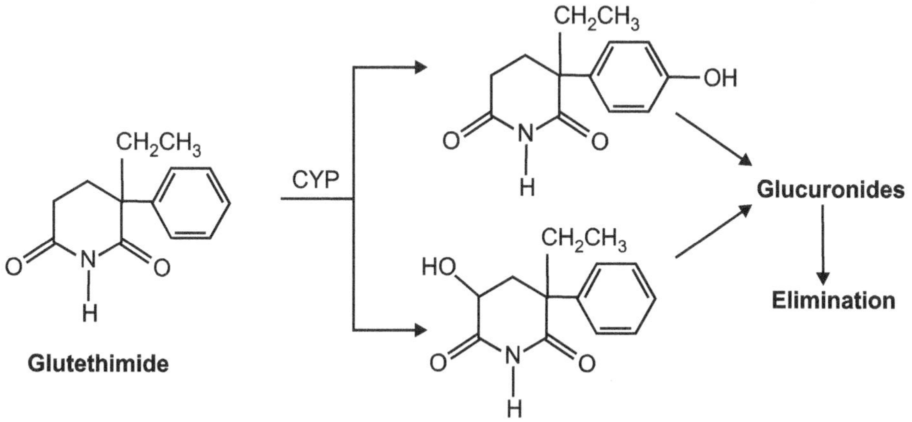

Metabolism/Execretion: Glutethimide is a racemate; both isomers are hydroxylated and both hydroxylated metabolites are reported to be active as sedative. These metabolites are conjugated with glucuronic acid. The glucuronides pass into the enterohepatic circulation and are excreted in the urine (< 2% unchanged).

4.6.2 Alcohols and their Carbamate Derivatives

The very simple alcohol ethanol has a long history of use as a sedative and hypnotic. Its modes of action were described under the anesthetic heading and are said to apply to other alcohols. It is widely used in self-medication as a sedative-hypnotic. Because this use has so many hazards, it is seldom a preferred agent medically.

Ethchlorvynol:

Ethchlorvynol is 1-chloro-3-ethyl-1-penten-4-yn-3-ol. It is prepared from ethyl chlorovinyl ketone by following chemical reactions under strict anhydrous conditions.

Ethchlorvynol is a mild sedative–hypnotic with a quick onset and short duration of action ($t_{1/2}$ 5.6 hours). Because of its highly lipophilic character, it is extensively metabolized to its secondary alcohol (90%) prior to its excretion. It reportedly induces microsomal hepatic enzymes.

Properties: Ethchlorvynol is a yellow coloured liquid with characteristic odour. It is light.

Uses: Ethchlorvynol is a short term hypnotic used to treat insomnia. It has rapid onset, short duration of action sensitive drug hence should be protected from light.

Ethchlorvynol

Meprobamate:

Chemistry: Meprobamate is 2-methyl-2-propyl trimethylene dicarbamate. Meprobamate is propanediol derivative.

Properties: Meprobamate is an odourless, white coloured crystalline aggregate with bitter taste. It is insoluble in water but soluble in alcohol and slightly soluble in ether.

Step 1: Meprobamate is prepared by condensing 2-methyl 2-n-propyl-1,3-propanediol with phosgene at 0°C to get chloroformate diester.

Step 2: The chloroformate diester is subjected to ammonolysis to form meprobamate.

Meprobamate

Uses: Meprobamate is used to induce sleep in anxiety and tensive patients. It also possesses anticonvulsant and muscle relaxant properties.

4.6.3 Aldehydes and their Derivatives

Paraldehyde:

Chemistry: Paraldehyde is a cyclic trimer of acetaldehyde. Chemically paraldehyde is 2,4,6-trimethyl-1, 3, 5-trioxane. It is prepared by condensing 3 molecules of acetaldehyde in the presence of small quantities of a catalyst (SO_2 or HCl or $ZnCl_2$).

Properties: Paraldehyde is available as colourless or pale yellow colour liquid. It has strong characteristic odour and is soluble in water. Paraldehyde should be stored in airtight, light protected containers.

Acetaldehyde

Paraldehyde

Uses: Paraldehyde is one of the oldest hypnotic. It is used as a hypnotic and sedative.

Triclofos Sodium:

Triclofos is 2,2,2-trichloroethylhydrogen orthophosphate, which occurs as its sodium salt. Triclofos sodium is hygroscopic, white colored, water soluble powder. Triclofos is used as hypnotic and sedative.

$$Cl-\underset{\underset{Cl}{|}}{\overset{\overset{Cl}{|}}{C}}-CH_2-O-\underset{\underset{OH}{|}}{\overset{\overset{O}{||}}{P}}-O^-\ Na^+$$

(B) ANTIPSYCHOTICS

4.7 INTRODUCTION

Psychoactive or psychotropic drugs are also known as tranquilizers. These drugs are used in the treatment of psychiatric disorders i.e. abnormalities of mental function. The psychoactive drugs render the patient calm and peaceful by reducing agitation and anxiety. Psychoactive drugs does not cure mental disorders but the available drugs do control most symptomatic manifestations and behavioural deviances, facilitate the patient's tendency toward remission and improve the capacity of patient for social, occupational, and familial adjustment. The primary characteristic feature of these drugs is that they alter the mental state and behaviour in a predictable way. Tranquilizers fall into two main classes, major and minor. **Major tranquilizers**, which are also known as antipsychotic agents, or neuroleptics, are so called because they are used to treat major states of mental disturbance in schizophrenics and other psychotic patients. **Minor tranquilizers**, which are also known as antianxiety agents or anxiolytics, are used to treat milder states of anxiety and tension in healthy individuals or people with less serious mental disorders.

4.8 PHENOTHIAZINE

Introduction

Phenothiazine derivatives are chemically characterized by a lipophilic fused tricyclic system (the phenothiazine nucleus) linked through the nitrogen atom of the central ring to a hydrophilic aminoalkyl substituent (the tertiary basic side chain).

First synthesized in 1950, chlorpromazine was the first drug developed with specific antipsychotic action, and would serve as the prototype for the phenothiazine class of drugs

Phenothiazines act exclusively on specific postsynaptic receptors and block the post synaptic dopamine receptors. They work on the positive symptoms of psychosis such as hallucinations, delusions, disorganized speech, looseness of association, and bizarre behavior. Phenothiazines are chemically constituted by a lipophilic, linearly fused tricyclic system having a hydrophilic basic amino alkyl chain. The following is the general structure of antipsychotic drugs.

Mechanism of Action:

Evidence supports the hypothesis that the etiology of psychotic disorders lies in neurochemical defects of ***dopaminergic*** and ***serotonergic*** pathways in the brain. This hypothesis is supported by the fact that the primary pharmacological action of antipsychotic agents is antagonism of dopamine and/or serotonin receptor in the CNS.

Physicochemical Properties:

1. The phenothiazine heterocycle having a high degree of lipophilicity on these antipsychotics, which is balanced (solubility) by the cationized (at physiologic pH) amine function

2. H_2O solubility of the antipsychotics phenothiazines is increased for oral dosage formulation bytreatment with an acid

3. The phenothiazines possess two potentially basic functional groups:

➢ The N^{10}-amine which is very weakly basic ($pK_b > 10$) because of the electron withdrawing effects of the 2 benzene rings attached to it and is not appreciably cationized at physiological pH.

➢ The side chain tertiary amine function which confers strong organic basicity on the antipsychotic phenothiazines.

Structural Activity Relationship of Phenothiazine:

Phenothiazines are the derivatives of phenothiazine tricyclic hetetocyclic moiety. The central ring possesses nitrogen and sulphur heteroatoms.

Modification of the Alkyl Side Chain:

➢ The maximum antipshycotic property or potency is observed when nitrogen of phenothiazine being present on the side chain nitrogen are connected by 3-carbon between two 'N' atoms, because it resembles with that of the dopamine (DA) structure.

Promazine　　　　　　　　　　　**Dopamine**

➢ Increase or decrease in the length of the alkyl side chain from 3 carbons, decreases the activity. Shortening of the chain to 2-carbons results in a change in receptor affinity from DA to CNS histamine receptors. Molecules with 2 carbon side chain are the antagonist.

(Anti-histaminic)

➢ Introduction of methyl group at α-carbon decreases antipsychotic activity and produces imipramine like activity. Substitution at the β-position of the side chain with small group like methyl will decrease the antipsychotic potency but increase the anti-histaminic activity.

➢ But substitution at β-position of the side chain with larger group decreases both anti-psychotic and anti-histaminic activity. Substitution at γ-position increases anti-cholinergic activity and decreases dopaminergic antagonism.

ADR- EPS (Extra pyrimidal syndrome)

Amino Group Modification:

➢ 3° nitrogen shows maximum potency whereas 2° and 1° show reduced or abolished activity. i.e. **3° > 2° >1°**.

Promazine

➢ N-alkylation with more than one carbon atom decreases activity. Activity is increased when dimethyl amino group is replaced by pyrrolidinyl, morpholinyl or thiomorpholinyl groups. i.e., Structural modification of the side chain amine function yields three anti-psychotic phenothiazine subclasses.

Prochlorperazine　　　　　**Chloropromazine (Aliphatic)**

➢ Introduction of –OH, CH_3, CH_3CH_3OH at C-4 of piperazine results in increased activity.

Fluphenazine

➢ Quaternary amino group contain molecule as inactive because they are positively charged and cannot pass or cross blood brain barrier. Pharmacologic/therapeutic profiles of these three classes of antipsychotics differ as follows:

Antipsychotic potency: Piperazines > Piperidines > Aliphatics.

EPS frequency: Piperazines > Piperidines > Aliphatics.

Sedation: Aliphatics = Piperidines > Piperazines.

Hypotension: Aliphatics > Piperidines > Piperazines.

Phenothiazine Ring Modification:

➢ Presence of electron withdrawing group at C-2 position on phenyl ring increases antipsychotic activity. The order of potency is in position 2 > 3 > 4 > 1.

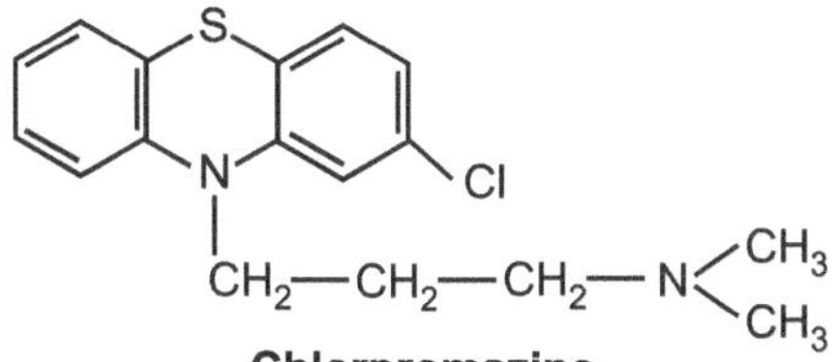

Chlorpromazine

➢ Potency of various groups increases in the following order,

OH < H < CN < CH$_3$< Cl < CF$_3$

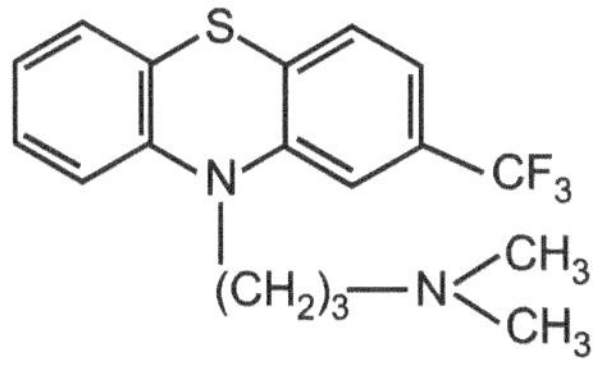

Triflupromazine

➢ Disubstitution or trisubstitution of the C-2 substituted drugs results in harmful potency. CF$_3$ is more potent than Cl but EPS (Extra pyramidal symptoms) appears. Hence chlorpromazine is much used than triflupromazine. Substitution at C-1 position decreases antipsychotic activity because it interferes with the bending of the side chain. (i.e., alkyl). Substitution at C-4 position may also interfere with S-binding to receptor. Multiple disubstitution on the ring system decreases potency (disubstitution on phenothiazine ring decreases neuroleptic potency).

➢ Conversion of ring sulphur into sulphoxide or sulphone decreases activity.

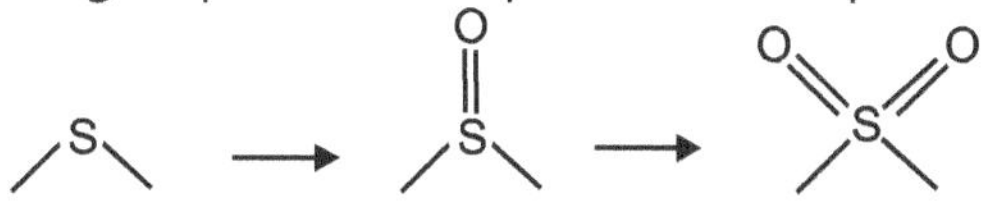

Ring Sulphur   Sulfoxide   Sulfone

4.9 PHENOTHIAZINE DERIVATIVE

Promazine Hydrochloride

Chemistry: Promazine hydrochloride is a phenothiazine derivative. Chemically it is 10-[3-(dimethylamino)-propyl] phenothiazine. Promazine is prepared by condensing 3-chloro-N, N dimethylpropylamine with phenothiazine in the presence of sodium hydride.

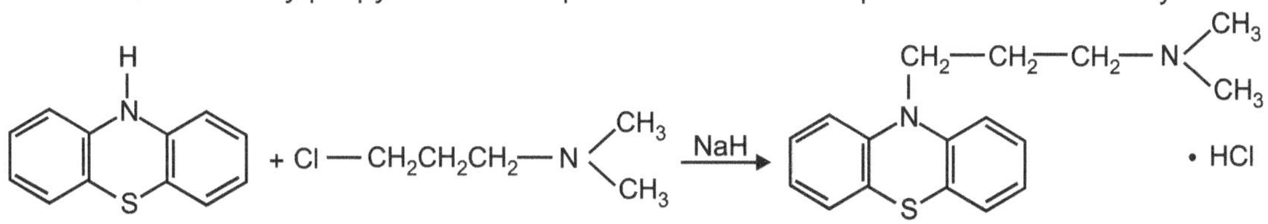

Promazine hydrochloride

Properties: Promazine is available as a hydrochloride salt. Promazine HCl is white or slightly yellow crystalline powder, and is freely soluble in water and chloroform. It should be protected from air.

Uses: Promazine has antipsychotic properties and also used to control nausea and vomiting.

Chlorpromazine Hydrochloride

Chemistry: Chlorpromazine hydrochloride is a phenothiazine derivative and has a chemical formula of 2-chloro-10-[3-(-dimethylamino) propyl] phenothiazine monohydro-chloride. Chlorpromazine is synthesized by cyclization of 3-chlorodiphenylamine with sulphur in the presence of small amount of iodine as a catalyst.

3-Chlorodiphenylamine

Chloropromazine hydrocloride

Properties: Chlorpromazine hydrochloride is an odourless, white crystalline powder. It is freely soluble in water, alcohol, chloroform and insoluble in ether and benzene. It decomposes on exposure to air and light, hence it should be stored in airtight containers and protect from light.

Mechanism of Action: Chlorpromazine blocks dopamine at D_2 receptor sites in the mesolimbic medullary chemoreceptor trigger zone areas of the brain. It causes inhibitory post-synaptic effects by reducing the flow of dopamine as the dopaminergic ion channels are closed.

Uses: Chlorpromazine is used in the management of psychotic conditions. It also controls excitement, aggression and agitation. It has antiemetic, antipruritic, anti-histaminic and sedative properties.

Side Effects:

Extra pyramidal symptoms, hypertension, orthostatic hypotension, blurred vision, dry mouth, anorexia, nausea, vomiting, constipation, diarrhoea, weight gain, impotence, amenorrhea, photosensitivity.

Trifluopromazine

Chemistry: Trifluopromazine is a fluorinated phenothiazine derivative. Chemically, triflupromazine is 10-[3-(dimethylamino)propyl]-2-(trifluoromethyl) phenothiazine. Trifluo-promazine is synthesized by condensing 2-(trifluoromethyl) phenothiazine with (3-chloropropyl) dimethylamine in dry benzene in the presence of sodamide.

2-(Trifluoromethyl)-phenothiazine

Triflupromazine

Properties: Promazine is available as hydrochloride salt. Promazine HCl is white or slightly yellow crystalline powder, and is freely soluble in water and chloroform. It should be protected from air.

Uses: Promazine has antipsychotic properties. It is also used to control nausea and vomiting.

Thioridazine Hydrochloride:

Thioridazine hydrochloride is a piperidine typical antipsychotic drug belonging to the phenothiazine derivative. Chemically, 2-ethyl-10-(2-(1-methylpiperidin-2-yl)ethyl)-10H-phenothiazine. R enantiomer has higher affinity for D_2 receptor.

Thioridazine hydrochloride

Uses: It is used in the treatment of schizophrenia and psychosis.

Thioridazine can cause life-threatening side effect of irregular heart beat that may cause sudden death.

Piperacetazine Hydrochloride:

Piperacetazine hydrochloride is a piperzine antipsychotic prodrug belonging to the phenothiazine derivative used for the treatment of schizophrenia. In veterinary practice greatest value of piperacetazine in anti-psychotic and and behaviour changes. Chemically, 1-(10-(3-(4-(2-hydroxyethyl)piperazin-1-yl)propyl)-10H-phenothiazin-2-yl)ethanone.

Piperacetazine hydrochloride

Prochlorperazine:

Chemistry: Prochlorperazine is a phenothiazine derivative associated with piperazine. Chemically, prochlorperazine is 3-chloro-10-[3-(4-methyl-1-piperazinyl) phenothiazine. It occurs as maleate and mesylate salts. Prochlorperazine is prepared by refluxing 1-(3-chloro propyl)-4-methylpiperazine with 2-chlorophenothiazine in the presence of sodamide in toluene.

2-Chlorophenothiazine

Prochlorperazine

Properties: Prochlorperazine is a pale yellow coloured, viscous liquid and is very slightly soluble in water but freely soluble in alcohol.

Uses: Prochlorperazine is an antipsychotic and tranquilizing agent. It is used to treat various psychiatric disorders such as schizophrenia, mania, involution psychoses, senile and tonic psychoses. It also has antiemetic properties.

Trifluperazine Hydrochloride:

Chemistry: Trifluperazine hydrochloride is a fluorinated phenothiazine derivative. Chemically, 2-(trifluoromethyl)-10-(3-(4-methylpiperazin-1-yl)propyl)-10H-phenothiazine.

Trifluperazine hydrochloride

Uses: Triflupromazine is used to treat psychotic disorders, schizophrenia, anxiety and other conditions.

Fluorobutyrophenone:

Flurobutyrophenone

The fluorobutyrophenones belong to a much-studied class of compounds, with many compounds possessing high antipsychotic activity. They were obtained by structure variation of the analgesic drug meperidine by substitution of the N-methyl by butyrophenone moiety to produce the butyrophenone analogue which has similar activity as chlorpromazine.

Meperidine　　　　　　**Butyrophenone analog**

Structure-activity Relationships of Fluorobutyrophenones:

The 4-aryl piperidino moiety is superimposable on the 2-phenylethylamino moiety of dopamine and, accordingly, could promote affinity for D_2 receptors. The long N-alkyl substituent could help promote affinity and produce antagonistic activity.

The structural requirements for antipsychotic activity in the group are well worked out. General features are expressed in the following structure.

➢ Para-F or similar electronegative substituent (e.g. CF_3) provides maximal potency is seen when with an aromatic ring.

➢ X = C=O (ketone) for optimal activity. Carbonyl group of butyrophenones is necessary for antipsychotic activity. Replacement of carbonyl group by functional groups such as X = C(H)OH or C(H)aryl structural feature yields therapeutically useful antipsychotics (e.g. Pimozide).

Pimozide

- ➢ Altering length or branching of the three-carbon chain linking keto and amino group decreases antipsychotic activity i.e. Propylene bridge is required for antipsychotic properties. Shortening or lengthening or branching of propylene bridge decreases antipsychotic activity.
- ➢ Terminal basic amine function may vary in structure but is usually incorporated in a 6-membered heterocyclic ring.
- ➢ AR is an aromatic ring attached directly to or separated by one atom from position 4 of the six membered ring.
- ➢ The Y group is variable and can enhance activity (Y = OH in haloperidol).

Fluorobutyrophenone Derivatives:

Haloperidol:

Chemistry: Haloperidol is a butyrophenone derivative with antipsychotic properties that has also been found as effective in lowering levels of hyperactivity, agitation, and mania. It has chemical formula of 4-[4-(p-chlorophenyl)-4-hydroxypiperidino]-4'-fluorobutyro-phenone. Haloperidol is synthesized by condensing 4-(4-chlorophenyl-4-piperidinol with 4-chloro-4'-fluorobutyrophenone.

Haloperidol

The mechanism inhibitions the transport mechanism of cerebral monoamines, particularly by blocking the impulse transmission in dopaminergic neurons. Peak plasma levels of haloperidol reach within 2 to 6 hours of oral administration.

Uses: The compound is a potent antipsychotic useful in schizophrenia and in psychoses associated with brain damage. It is often chosen as the agent to terminate mania.

Risperidone:

Chemistry: Risperidone is a benzisoxazole derivative with high affinity for central serotonergic 5-HT$_2$, dopaminergic D$_2$ and adrenergic α_1-receptors *in-vivo*. HCl salt is used for oral formulation. schizophrenia and reduced EPS.

Risperidone

Droperidol:

Droperidol is a benzimidazolinone derivative of fluorobutyrophenones. Chemically, it is 1-{1-[3-(p-Fluorobenzoyl)propyl]-1,2,5,6-tetrahydro-4-pyridyl}-2-benzimidazolinone. It is used alone as a preanesthetic neuroleptic or as an antiemetic. Its most frequent use is in combination with the narcotic agent fentanyl preanesthetically. It is considered as a short-acting sedating butyrophenone and sometimes used in psychiatric emergencies as a sedative-neuroleptic.

Droperidol

Beta Amino Ketones:

Molindone hydrochloride:

Molindone hydrochloride is a dihydroindolone compound which is not structurally related to the phenothiazines, the butyrophenones or the thioxanthenes. Chemically, is 3-ethyl-6, 7-dihydro-2-methyl-5-(morpholinomethyl) indol-4 (5H)-one hydrochloride. It is a white to off-white crystalline powder, freely soluble in water and alcohol.

Molindone hydrochloride

Thiothixene: The thioxanthenes differ from the phenothiazines by the replacement of nitrogen in the central ring with a carbon-linked side chain fixed in space in a rigid structural configuration. An N,N-dimethyl sulfonamide functional group is bonded to the thioxanthene nucleus. Chemically, it is N,N-dimethyl-9-[3-(4-methyl-1-piperazinyl)-propylidene] thioxanthene-2-sulfonamide, *Z* isomer (cis isomer) is more active than *E* isomer (trans). They act as dopamine 2-antagonist Schizophrenia, other psychotic disorders and bipolar disorder. Psychotic symptoms can also improve within 1 week, but it may take several weeks for full effect on behaviour.

Thiothixene

Clozapine: Clozapine are dibenzazepines or dibenzodiazepine derivatives and first a typical antipsychotic agent. They show week D_2 blocking action but act as strong D_4 receptors and $5HT_2$ receptor.

Clozapine

Loxitane: Loxapine, a dibenzoxazepine compound, represents a subclass of tricyclic antipsychotic agent, chemically distinct from the thioxanthenes, butyrophenones, and phenothiazines. Chemically, it is 2-Chloro-11 (4-methyl-1-piperazinyl)dibenz[b,f][1,4] oxazepine. It is present in capsules as the succinate salt, and in the concentrate and parenteral primarily as the hydrochloride salt. It is used for the treatment of schizophrenia. The major pharmacological mode of action involves dopamine D_2 receptor antagonism, and to a lesser extent, blocking activity at D_1 receptors as well.

Benzamide

Sulpiride: Sulpiride are a typical antipsychotic benzamide derivatives. It is used in the management of the symptoms of schizophrenia. Chemically, sulpiride is a selective antagonist at dopamine D_2 and D_3 receptors thereby reduce positive symptoms of psychosis.

Sulpiride can be synthesized from 5-aminosulfosalicylic acid. Methylating this with dimethylsulfate gives 2-methoxy-5-aminosulfonylbenzoic acid, which is transformed into an amide using 2-aminomethyl-1-ethylpyrrolidine as the amine component and carbonyl diimidazole (CDI) as a condensing agent.

5-aminosulfosalicylic acid

Methoxy-5-aminosulfonyl benzoic acid

Sulpiride

(C) ANTICONVULSANTS

4.10 INTRODUCTION

Epilepsy is a common but serious brain disorder. It is universal, with no age, sex, geographical, social class or racial boundaries. Epilepsy imposes a large economic burden on health care systems of countries. There is also a hidden burden associated with stigma and discrimination against the patient and even his/her family in the community, workplace, school and home. Many patients with epilepsy suffer severe emotional distress, behavioural disorders and extreme social isolation.

4.11 WHAT IS EPILEPSY?

Epilepsy can be defined as "the occurrence of transient paroxysms of excessive or uncontrolled discharges of neurons, which may be due to a number of different causes leading to epileptic seizures". The actual presentation or manifestation differs among individuals, depending upon the location of the origin of the epileptic discharges in the brain and their spread. A person should only be diagnosed as having "epilepsy" if there are recurrent manifestations; the first episode of a seizure is called a "single seizure" and not epilepsy.

An epileptic seizure is an event in which an individual is not aware of the surroundings, either completely or partially. Various motor movements, such as shaking of limbs; sensory phenomenon, such as electric shock-like sensation over a specific area; behavioural experiences, such as fear or confusion or autonomic disturbances such as excessive secretion of saliva or bladder/bowel incontinence could occur in association with this altered sensorium. Usually it is very brief, lasting from a few seconds to minutes. Only in very rare cases will it be continuous, resulting in "status epilepticus", i.e. a seizure lasting more than 30 minutes or recurrent seizures without the individual regaining consciousness between attacks.

4.12 CLASSIFICATION OF EPILEPTIC SEIZURES

Epilepsy can broadly be divided into two categories: idiopathic where there is no known cause, and secondary seizures where there is known cause. Seizures can be either generalized or partial (or focal). In generalized seizures, both halves of the brain are simultaneously affected. In partial seizures, the abnormal electrical discharge starts from a focus in one side of the brain. Later, this may spread to the other side. This spread is called secondary generalization.

Generalized Seizures: In generalized seizures, patients suddenly stop what they are doing, the eyes and head turn to one side and the body becomes stiff. This is usually followed by several jerks of the hands and legs, groaning and frothing from the mouth. During the episode, the tongue may be bitten or severe injury can result from a fall or an accident. Sometimes the patient may pass urine or stools. The body relaxes after a few minutes and the patient sleeps for a variable period. The patient is completely unaware of the seizure. Such seizures can also occur in sleep.

Generalized seizures consist of many different seizure types, of which the primary generalized tonic-clonic seizure (GTCS) is the most common.

Tonic-clonic seizure: In a generalized tonic-clonic seizure the patient loses consciousness, falls down, sometimes with a scream, and develops a generalized stiffness (the tonic phase). Breathing stops, as all the muscles of the trunk are in spasm, and the patient becomes cyanotic, the head is retracted, the arms flexed and the legs extended. After a while, this tonic phase is followed by the clonic phase, when the muscles alternately contract and relax, resulting in clonic movements. During this jerking the patient might bite his tongue, pass urine, or sometimes stool. The clonic phase may last several minutes. When all the jerking stops and the patient regain consciousness, he may feel very tired and have a headache and confusion. He has no memory of what happened, and may find himself on the floor in a strange position. Often he falls into a deep sleep. The frequency of the seizure may vary from one a day to one a month or once a year, or even once every few years. Either the tonic phase or the clonic phase can predominate in the seizure. Generalized tonic-clonic seizures can also occur due to secondary generalization in partial epilepsies.

Clonic seizures: These seizures are generalized seizures, where the tonic component is not present, only repetitive clonic jerks (clonic jerks are repetitive rhythmic flexing and stretching of limbs). When the frequency of jerks diminishes the amplitude of the jerks does not diminish.

Tonic seizures: Tonic seizures are sudden sustained muscle contractions, fixing the limbs in some strained position. There is immediate loss of consciousness. Often there is deviation of eyes and head towards one side, sometimes rotation of the whole body.

Absence seizures: These are short periods of loss of consciousness lasting only a few seconds (not more than half a minute). They are of sudden onset, there are usually no, or only minimal motor manifestations. There is a blank stare, brief upward rotation of the eyes and an interruption of ongoing activity. The child is unresponsive when spoken to. It is suddenly over, and the child continues what he was doing before the seizure. The child has no memory of these seizures.

Myoclonic seizures: These seizures consist of sudden, brief, shock-like muscle contractions, either occurring in one limb, or more widespread and bilateral. They may be single jerks, or jerks repeated over longer periods. They are often seen in combination with other seizure types occurring in special epileptic syndromes.

Partial Seizures: Partial seizures are divided into two groups, simple partial seizures where consciousness is maintained and complex partial seizures where there is an impairment of consciousness.

Simple partial seizures: In simple partial seizures, some patients may experience either motor or sensory phenomena. Such seizures arise from a specific area of the brain, with the patient being fully or partly aware of the event. In motor seizures, the focus is in the primary motor cortex. There are twitchings, starting in a distal part of the extremity, or in the face. The twitching may remain localised, or spread up the whole extremity and even become completely generalized to involve the whole body. Sensory seizures have their focus in the post-central gyrus (primary sensory cortex). There might be feelings of tingling, pins and needles, cold or heat, or numbness of a limb. Sometimes there may be strange feelings with visual signs, or hearing or smelling sensations. Autonomic seizures are associated with foci in the temporal lobe. There maybe: a sensation rising from the epigastrium to the throat, palpitations, sweating or flushing. The psychic symptoms may consist of changes in mood, memory, or thought (thinking). There may be distorted perceptions (time, space, or person) or problems with language. Structured hallucinations could occur (music, scenes). These simple partial seizures are usually only recognized as epileptic seizures when they develop into generalized seizures

Complex partial seizures: Here the patient has impaired consciousness, but NOT complete loss of consciousness. He is slightly aware of what is going on, but he cannot respond to anything, neither can he change his behaviour during an attack. The seizure usually starts with an aura which can be of many types such as, a strange feeling in the stomach rising up to the throat and head, or a sensation of light, smell, sound or taste or with changes in perception, e.g., of time (time seems to pass too slowly or too fast), of light or sound or space. Sometimes the seizure occurs with hallucinations or with psychomotor symptoms such as automatisms e.g., pulling at the clothes, chewing, lip smacking, or repeated aimless movements.

There are different ways to treat the epilepsy by different mechanism:

- By inhibiting Na^+ channels (reduction of electrical excitability of cell membranes).

  Ex: Phenytoin, Carbamazepine, Valproate, Lamotrigine Phenytoin).

- By inhibiting GABA transaminase enzyme (Enhancement of GABA-ergic action).

  Ex: Phenobarbital, Benzodiazepines, Vigabatrin, Gabapentin).

- By inhibition of calcium channel function (T-type calcium channels).

  Ex: Ethosuximide, Gabapentin.

However, it is believed that the anticonvulsants suppress seizures by depressing the cerebral (motor) cortex of the brain, thereby raising the threshold of the central nervous system (CNS) to convulsive stimuli. Therefore, the person is less likely to undergo seizures.

4.13 CLASSIFICATION OF ANTICONVULSANTS

The anticonvulsants are classified as:

- ➢ **Barbiturates:** Phenobarbitone, Methabarbital.
- ➢ **Hydantoins:** Phenytoin*, Mephenytoin, Ethotoin
- ➢ **Oxazolidine diones:** Trimethadione, Paramethadione

➢ **Succinimides:** Phensuximide, Methsuximide, Ethosuximide

➢ **Urea and monoacylureas:** Phenacemide, Carbamazepine

➢ **Benzodiazepines:** Clonazepam.

➢ **Miscellaneous:** Primidone, Valproic acid, Gabapentin, Felbamate.

Barbiturates:

It has a pyrimidine derivative it is usually depicted as the cyclical ureide of malonic acid in either the keto or enol form. Barbituric acid is hypnotically inert but the introduction of organic substituents at position 5 endows the resultant drugs with the ability to depress consciousness. Diethylbarbituric acid or barbitone is the first sedative barbiturate. Barbitone was popular as a hypnotic for many years but it was too long-lasting for general use. Phenobarbitone was the next drug to be developed.

Long-acting barbiturates such as phenobarbital (Luminal) and mephobarbital (Mebaral) are prescribed for two main reasons. When taken at bedtime, they help treat insomnia. When taken during the day, they have sedative effects that can aid in the treatment of tension and anxiety. These same effects have been found helpful in the treatment of convulsive conditions like epilepsy. Phenobarbital has also been used in the treatment of delirium tremens during alcohol detoxification, although benzodiazepines have a more favorable safety profile and are more often used.

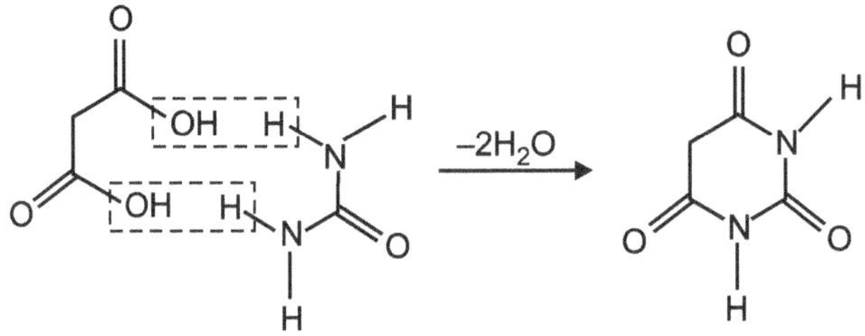

Mechanism of Action of Barbiturates:

Barbiturates act on GABA receptors in central nervous system and increase the GABAergic inhibition of central nervous system.

Structural Activity Relationship:

Structural feature and structural activity relationship of antiepileptic drugs, the molecules should have at least one aryl or lipophilic units, one or two hydrogen acceptor-donor atoms and an electron donor atom in a unique spatial arrangement to be recommended for antiepileptic activity, for example mephobarbitone, ethotoin, gabapentin and zonisamide etc. are characterized as their structural elements. These agents exert their action by different mechanisms. They include an enhancement of the GABA-ergic neurotransmission, effects on neuronal voltage-gated Na^+ and/or Ca^{2+} channels.

Structure: N-H or N-Methyl and C-5 side chains consisting of two ethyl groups, or an ethyl and phenyl group.

General Properties: Relatively low lipophilicity and low plasma protein binding.

Phenobarbital (Phenobarbitone):

Phenobarbital is the oldest currently available AEDs. Although it has long been considered one of the safest of the AED, the use of other medications with lesser sedative effects has been urged. The barbiturates are considered as the drugs of choice for the treatment of seizures only in infants.

Phenobarbital

The four barbituric acid derivatives are clinically useful as AEDs are phenobarbitone (PBT), mephobarbital, metharbital, and primidone. The metharbital is methylated barbital and mephobarbital is methylated PBT; both are demethylated. Chemically phenobarbital is 5-ethyl-5-phenyl-1H, 3H, 5H-pyrimidine-2,4,6-trione and first antiepileptic drug ever developed. Antiepileptic action is seen in most of barbiturates, however, phenobarbital shows antiepileptic action in lower concentrations with acceptable degree of sedation.

- Phenobarbital is orally administered in the treatment of grandmal epilepsy.

- It is less effective in the treatment of petitmal and psychomotor epilepsies. The injectable form of the drug is used to treat other types of convulsions.

Barbiturates with phenytoin show better antiepileptics (which are better tolerable especially with regard on sedative effects).

Mechanism of Action of Barbiturates:

Phenobarbital (PBT) suppresses high-frequency recurring firing in neurons in culture by an action on Na^+ ion conductance. Barbiturates block some Ca^{2+} ion currents (L-type and N-type). The PBT binds to an allosteric regulatory site on the GABA-BZD receptor, and it improved the GABA receptor-mediated current by extending the openings of the Cl^- channels. The PBT also blocks excitatory responses stimulated by glutamate, mainly those mediated by activation of the AMPA receptor. Both the enrichment of GABA-mediated inhibition and the decline of glutamate mediated excitation are seen with therapeutically applicable concentrations of PBT. The PBT is valuable in the therapy of partial seizures and generalized tonic-clonic seizures, even though the drug is often tried for all seizure type, particularly when attacks are complicated to manage.

Adverse Effects:

The most common adverse effects associated with phenobarbital are sedation (although a degree of tolerance develops), dizziness, drowsiness, ataxia (lack of muscula and nystagmus (a rapid involuntary movement of the eyeball).

Methabarbital:

Phenobarbital's success led to the development of other barbiturates as subsequent AEDs, including the *N*-methyl barbituric acid derivatives mephobarbital (N-methylphenobarbital), introduced in 1932. Like phenobarbital, both mephobarbital are water-insoluble weak acids with pK$_a$ values of 7.8 and 8.5, respectively. The introduction of the *N*-methyl group into the phenobarbital molecule breaks the symmetric axis possessed by barbituric acid or phenobarbital. Consequently, unlike phenobarbital, mephobarbital is a chiral compound containing one asymmetric carbon atom at position 5 of the molecule. It has been used clinically as racemic mixtures (equal parts of (R)- and (S)-enantiomers). Mephobarbital metabolism is stereoselective with (R)-methylphenobarbital being metabolized by cytochrome P450 (CYP)2C19-mediated aromatic hydroxylation (a genetic polymorphism-susceptible metabolic pathway coregulated by mephenytoin hydroxylation), whereas (S)-methylphenobarbital undergoes CYP2D6-mediated demethylation to form phenobarbital. In contrast to phenobarbital, mephobarbital is currently not widely used.

Methabarbital

Hydantoins:

Hydantoins are cyclic monoacylureas. They possess imidazoline-2,4-dione heterocyclic system and are structurally related to barbiturates, differing in lacking the 6-oxo moiety. Hydantoins are weakly acidic than barbiturates. Thus aqueous solutions of sodium salts provide strongly alkaline solutions. Clinically useful hydantoin possess an aryl substituent at the 5-position and derivatives possessing of lower alkyl substituents have antiabsence activity.

Structural Activity Relationship:

- A phenyl or other aromatic substitutions at C$_5$ is essential for the activity.
- Alkyl substitutions at position C$_5$ may contribute to sedation, a property which is absent in phenytoin.

Mephenytoin   **Phenytoin**

- Among other hypnotics 1,3-disubstituted hydantoins exhibit activity against chemically induced convulsion. While it remains ineffective against electric shock induced convulsion.

- A clinically useful hydantoin possess an aryl substituent at the 5-position.

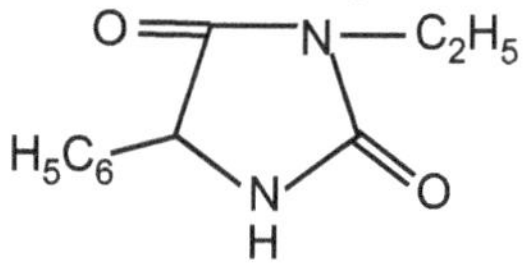

Ethotoin

Phenytoin:

The derivatives of hydantoin (imidazolidine-2,4-dione) are well known and clinically widely used in the therapy of epilepsy and cardiac arrhythmias. Phenytoin (5,5-diphenylhydantoin), one of the oldest anticonvulsants, is very effective in controlling a variety of seizure disorders, chemically 5,5-diphenylimidazolidine-2,4-dione. It is used to control certain type of seizures, and to treat and prevent seizures. It works by decreasing abnormal electrical activity in the brain. These effects are due to a selective block of high frequency neuronal activity. The drug targets the neuronal voltage sensitive sodium channels (NVSC) to reproduce the normal ion potential and is known to block the release of neurotransmitters, such as serotonin and norepinephrine. At an appropriate level, it inhibits monoamine oxidase activity and tends to alter the membrane potential. Phenytoin is used alone or in combination with phenobarbital in the treatment of grand mal and psychomotor epilepsy.

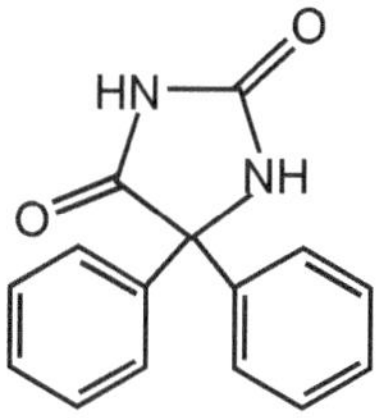

Synthesis:

5,5-diphenylimidazolidinedione is synthesized in two different ways. The first involves a base catalyzed addition of urea to benzil followed by a benzilic acid rearrangement (1,2 phenyl migration) to form the desired product.

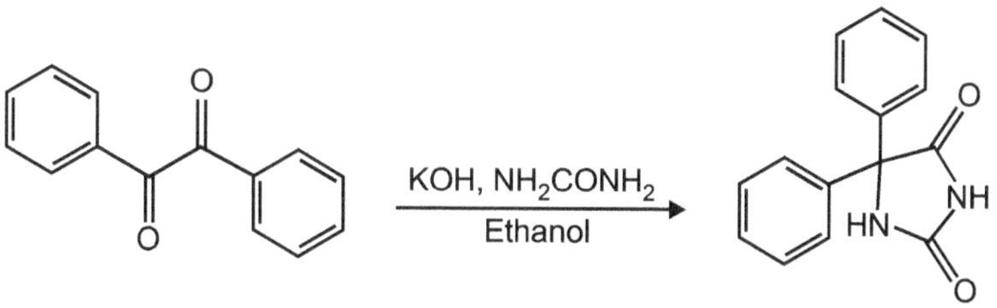

$$\text{KOH, NH}_2\text{CONH}_2 \xrightarrow{\text{Ethanol}}$$

Adverse Effects:

Adverse effects associated with phenytoin include ataxia, nystagmus and slurred speech.

Metabolism of Phenytoin:

The principal metabolic pathway of phenytoinin human is aromatic hydroxylation.

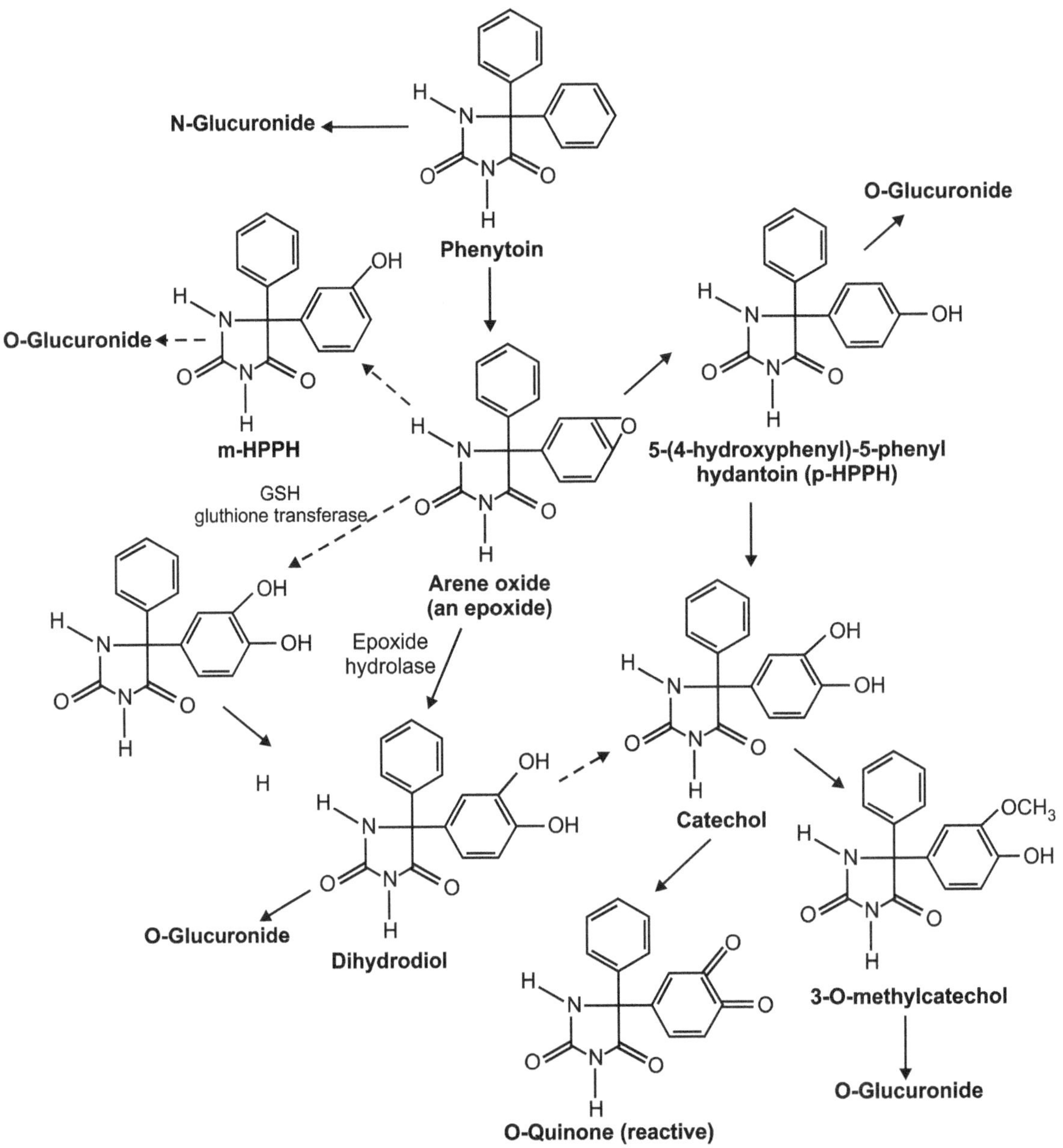

Mephenytoin:

Mephenytoin is a compound belonging to the phenylhydantoins (hydantoin derivative) compound containing an imidazolidinedione moiety substituted by a phenyl group. Mephenytoin is known to target sodium channel protein type 5 subunit alpha. Cytochrome P450 2C19, Cytochrome P450 2C8, Cytochrome P450 2C9, Cytochrome P450 2B6, Cytochrome P450 1A2, and Cytochrome P450 2D6 are known to metabolize mephenytoin.. Chemically it is ethyl-3-methyl-5-phenylimidazolidine-2,4-dione.

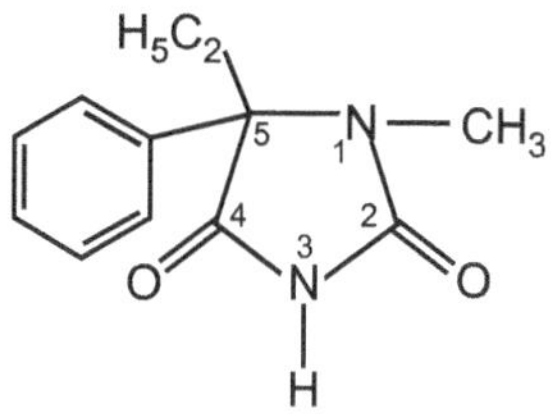

Mephenytoin

They have a marked anticonvulsive potency and are effective in grand mal seizure, focal epilepsy, and also in the case of status epilepticus without showing sedative-hypnotic properties.

Mechanism of Action:

The mechanism of action of mephenytoin is to block voltage-dependent neuronal sodium channels, and therefore limit repetitive firing of action potentials i.e. reduces the maximal activity of brain stem centers responsible for the tonic phase of tonic-clonic (grand mal) seizures.

Synthesis: Mephenytoin is prepared by the following steps:

- In the first step cyanoethylphenyl acetamide is prepared from cyanophenyl acetamide by treatment with sodium ethoxide and ethyliodide.

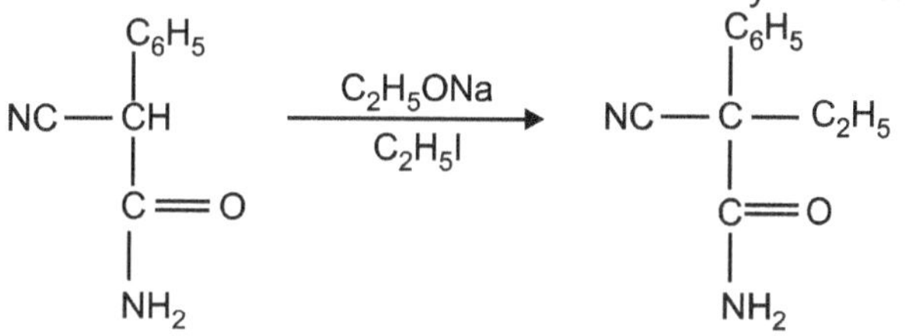

- The product obtained by oxidation with alkaline hypobromite solution converts cyano group of cyanoethylphenyl acetamide to amide group, which isomerizes and cyclised spontaneously.

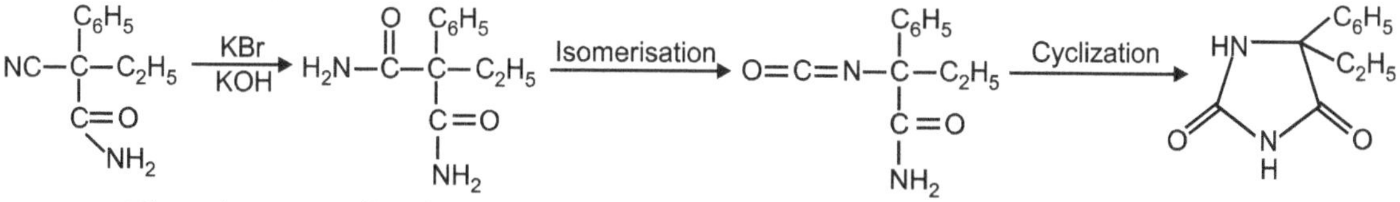

- The above cyclized product (5-ethyl 5-phenyl hydantoin) yield mephenytoin by methylation of the nitrogen atom (which is present between two carbonyl group) with methyl sulfate or methyliodide.

Oxazolidinediones:

Structural Activity Relationship:

Replacement of the –NH group at position-1 of the hydontoin system with oxygen atom yields the oxazolidinediones-2,4-dione system.

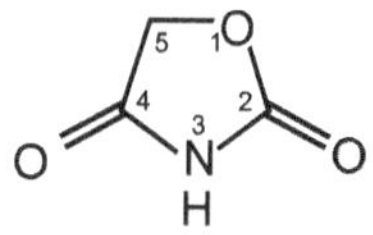

- Nature of the substitution on C-5 is essential for antiepileptic activity. Lower alkyl substitution towards anti-petitmal activity while acyl substituents towards anti-grandmal activity.
- The N-alkyl substituent does not alter or afford the activity because clinically used agents undergo metabolism to produce N-dealkylation compounds.

Trimethadione:

Trimethadione, the first oxazolidinedione, was introduced in 1945 and drug of choice for absence seizures until the introduction of succinimides in 1950s. The use of the oxazolidine-diones (trimethadione, paramethadione, and dimethadione) is now very limited. They contain an oxazolidine ring and have similar in structure to other antiepileptic agents introduced before 1960. These drugs are active against PTZ-induced seizures. Trimethadione is an oxazolidinedione derivative. Chemically it is 3,5,5-trimethyloxazolidine-2,4-dione.

Trimethadione raises the threshold for seizure discharges following repetitive thalamic stimulation. Its active metabolite dimethadione has the same effect on thalamic Ca^{2+} currents as ESM (reducing the T-type Ca^{2+} current). Thus, suppression of absence seizures is likely to depend on inhibiting the pacemaker action of thalamic neurons. The most common adverse effect is sedation and unusual adverse effect is hemeralopia, a glare effect in which visual adaptation is impaired. Accumulation of dimethadione causes a very mild metabolic acidosis and should not be used during pregnancy.

Synthesis:

Ethyl-α-hydroxy-α-methyl propionate is condensed with urea to yield 5, 5-dimethylox-azolidine-2, 4-dione, which on treatment with a strong base followed by methylation with methyl sulphate gives trimethadione.

Trimethadione

Paramethadione:

Paramethadione is 5-ethyl-3, 5-dimethyl oxazolidine-2, 4-dione. Structurally it is very closely related to trimethadione. Paramethadione is used in the treatment of absence seizures.

Succinimides:

Oxazolidinediones are toxic hence to replace them with less toxic drugs succinimides were introduced in 1951 as antiepileptics. Succinimide is a cyclic imide of succinic acid or 2,5-pyrrolidinedione and its derivatives had been known for their antiepileptic activity, particularly against petitmal type of epilepsy. The mechanism of action of succinimides has been postulated that succinimides enhances inhibitory processes in the brain, by inhibit T-type calcium channels and inhibit the three-cycle per second thalamic 'spike and wave' discharge in absence seizures. Succinimide anticonvulsants are mostly used to treat absence seizures.

Ethosuximide:

Ethosuximide is a succinimide anticonvulsant chemically designated as alpha-ethyl-alpha-methyl-succinimide i.e. (RS)-3-ethyl-3-methyl-pyrrolidine-2,5-dione), effective in the treatment of absence (petit mal) seizures.

Synthesis:

Methylethylketone and cyanoacetic ester, which undergo condensation. Then hydrogen cyanide is added. After acidic hydrolysis and decarboxylation of the synthesized dinitrile, 2-methyl-2-ethylsuccinic acid is formed. Reacting this product with ammonia gives the diammonium salt, and heterocyclization into ethosuximide takes place during subsequent heating.

Mechanism of Action:

Its ability to decrease low-threshold calcium currents in thalamic neurons by T-type Ca^{2+} channel inhibition thereby the frequency of epileptiform attacks is reduced, apparently by depression of the motor cortex and elevation of the threshold of the central nervous system to convulsive stimuli. It also inhibits Na^+/K^+ ATPase, depresses cerebral metabolic rate, and inhibits GABA aminotransferase.

Adverse Reactions:

Drowsiness, headache, fatigue, nausea, vomiting, idiosyncratic reactions and hematopoietic disturbances.

Phensuximide:

Phensuximide is a 2,5-pyrrolidinedione derivative. Chemically it is N-methyl-2-phenylsuccinimide. Phensuximide is a succinimide antiepileptic agent used to treat convulsions but it is reported to be less effective.

Phensuximide

Methsuximide:

Methosuximide is a succinimide antiepileptic drug. It is N, 2-dimethyl-2-phenylsuccinimide. Phensuximide and methsuximide are phenylsuccinimides that were developed before ethosuximide and used mainly as anti-absence drugs. Methsuximide has been used for partial seizures, it is more toxic, Phensuximide is less effective than ethosuximide. Unlike ESM, these two compounds have some activity against seizures. The desmethyl (N-desmethylmethsuccimide) metabolite of methsuximide exerts major anti-seizure effect.

Synthesis:

same steps as for phensuximide

Acetophenone　　**Ethyl cyanoacetate**　　　　**Methsuximide**

Urea and Monoacylureas:

Carbamazepine:

Carbamazepine is an azepine derivative possessing dibenzazepine nucleus. Carbamazepine is 5H-dibenzazepine-5-carboxamide.

Carbamazepine

Carbamazepine (CBZ) is closely related to imipramine and other tricyclic antidepressants, it is a tricyclic compound useful in management of bipolar depression. It was initially used for the therapy of trigeminal neuralgia but has established as useful antiepileptic agent as well. The ureide moiety ($-N-CO-NH_2$) present in the heterocyclic ring exist in CBZ. The mechanism of action of CBZ showed to be like as of Phenytoin. Like Phenytoin, CBZ exhibited activity against MES seizures. The CBZ blocks Na^+ channels at therapeutic concentration and inhibits high-frequency recurring firing in neurons. It also operates presynaptically to reduce synaptic transmissions. These effects possibly account for the anti-epileptic action of CBZ. It interacts with adenosine receptors and also inhibits uptake and release of norepinephrine from brain synaptosomes but does not control GABA uptake in brain. The indication suggested that the postsynaptic action of GABA can be potentiated by CBZ. It is the drug of choice for partial seizures, and may be used for treatment of generalized tonic-clonic seizures. It is also valuable in some patients with mania (bipolar disorder).

Synthesis: It is prepared by the following steps:

10,11-Dihydro-5H-dibenzazepine by acetylation followed by bromination with N-bromosuccinimide gives N-acetyl-11-bromo dibenzazepine.

Dehydrohalogenation of N- acetyl-11-bromo dibenzazepine followed by saponification with potassium hydroxide in ethanol leads to dibenzazepine.

Treatment of dibenzazepine with phosgene followed by heating with ammonia produces carbamazepine.

Uses: Carbamazepine is an antiepileptic drug used to control grandmal and focal seizures. It is also used in the treatment of trigeminal neuralgia and the treatment of manic depression.

Clonazepam:

Clonazepam is 5-(2-chlorophenyl)-3-dihydro-7-nitro-2H-1,4-benzodialzepin-2-one. Clonazepam is used in the treatment of grand mal epilepsy. It is the alternate drug for the treatment of petit mal in patients who fail to respond to ethosuximide therapy. It suppresses various types of status epilepticus seizures but because of its cardio-respiratory depressant effect.

Synthesis: p-Nitroaniline is treated with acetic anhydride to form an amide, thus protecting the amino group. Then followed by Friedel-Crafts acylation gives a diaryl ketone and removal of the amine protecting by hydrolysis of the amide in aqueous base gives the free amine. Then treatment of the amine with chloroacetyl chloride gives an α-chloroamide. Nucleophilic displacement of the primary chloride by ammonia gives a primary amine. The reaction of the primary amine with the nearby ketone gives an imine and closes the seven-membered ring of clonazepam.

Adverse Effect: The primary side effect associated with clonazepam is central nervous system depression.

Valproic Acid:

Mechanism of Action:

Block of voltage-gated sodium channels in neuronal membranes prevents Na^+ influx, which results in decreased axonal conductance by increasing the refractory period of the neuron and also inhibits GABA transaminase.

Use: Complex partial seizures as monotherapy and/or adjuvant, Simple and complex absence seizures, Myoclonic seizures, Migraine prophylaxis, Bipolar mania.

Synthesis:

Valproic acid may be synthesized from 4-heptanol by successive conversions to 4-bromoheptane with HBr, to 4-cyanoheptane with HCN and to 2-propyl pentanoic (valproic) acid by alkaline hydrolysis of 4-cyanoheptane.

4-Heptanol → (HBr) → **4-Bromoheptane** → (HCN) → **4-Cyanoheptane** → (Alkaline hydrolysis) → **Valproic acid**

Adverse Effects: Weight gain, pancreatitis, tremor, thrombocytopenia, headache, azoospermia, hirsutism, hair colour change.

Gabapentin:

Gabapentin containing primary amino and carboxyl groups, is better represented as an internal salt resulting from proton transfer from the acidic carboxyl group to the basic amino group.

Gabapentin → (Intramolecular acid/base reaction) → internal salt

Gabapentin is a derivative of GABA and effective against partial seizures. It is found to be more effective as an antiepileptic drug and appears not to act on GABA receptors. It may change GABA metabolism, its non-synaptic release, or its reuptake by GABA transporters. An enhancement in brain GABA concentration is seen. Gabapentin is carrying into the brain by the L-amino acid transporter. The drug also connected to the subunit of voltagesensitive Ca^{2+} channels. Gabapentin is active as an adjunct against partial and generalized tonic-clonic seizures. It is also effective in neuropathic pain and for post therapeutic neuralgia in adults. The most frequent adverse effects are somnolence, ataxia, dizziness, headache, and tremor.

Primidone:

Primidone is an antiepileptic agent related to barbiturates. Primidone is a diketone derived from hexahydropyrimidine. Chemically it is 5-ethyl-2, 3-dihydro-5-phenyl-4, 6-(1H, 5H)-pyrimidine dione.

Primidone (2-desoxyPBT) was metabolized in to phenobarbital and phenylethyl-malonamide (PEMA). All these three compounds are active against convulsions. Primidone is useful against partial seizures and generalized tonic-clonic seizures and may be more effective than phenobarbital. It was considered to be drug of choice for partial seizures, but the partial seizures in adults strongly suggest that CBZ and PHT are superior to primidone.

Synthesis: It is prepared from diethyl ethyl phenylmalonate by following steps:

Diethyl ethyl phenylmalonate is converted into its amide derivative by the action of ammonia.

Amide is refluxed with formamide to yield primidone.

Primidone

Felbamate:

The mechanism of action suggested that it is a NMDA receptor blockade *via* the glycine binding site. Felbamate has a half-life of 20 hrs and is metabolized by hydroxylation and conjugation; considerable amount of the drug is excreted unaffected in urine. When added to therapy with other antiepileptic drugs, felbamate enhanced plasma PHT and VLPA levels but reduces levels of CBZ. It is used in partial seizures and also active against the seizures that happen in Lennox-Gastaut syndrome.

Felbamate

QUESTIONS

1. What are sedatives and hypnotics? Classify them with suitable examples. Write the synthesis of chlordiazepoxide
2. Define sedatives and hypnotics. Explain the structural activity relationship of benzodiazepines.
3. Classify barbiturates with examples. Discuss the structural activity relationship of barbiturates. Outline the synthesis of phenobarbital.
4. Give the SAR of benzodiazepine derivatives. Outline the synthesis of Diazepam and Phenobarbital.
5. Outline the synthesis of Secobarbital or Phenobarbital.
6. Give the synthesis of glutethimide and meprobamate.
7. Write a note on barbiturate.
8. Discuss (a) Aldehydes and their derivatives (b) Amides and imides as useful sedatives and hypnotics.

DRUGS ACTING ON CENTRAL NERVOUS SYSTEM

◆ LEARNING OBJECTIVES ◆

After completing this unit, reader should be able to understand:

❖ To study the definition and ideal characteristics of general anaesthetics

❖ To understand the mechanism of action of general anaesthetic agents

❖ To study the classification of general anaesthetics in detail

❖ To learn the synthetic pathways of some selective general anaesthetics

❖ To learn about analgesic, classification and various opioid receptors

❖ To learn the structural activity relationship of morphine analogue

❖ To learn the synthetic pathways of some selective NSAIDs

5.1 GENERAL ANAESTHETICS

General anaesthetics are CNS depressants which cause partial or complete loss of consciousness, sense or pain. The effect is reversible and generally used to produce unconsciousness during painful surgeries.

General anaesthetics bring about descending depression of the CNS, starting with the cerebral cortex, the basal ganglia, the cerebellum and finally the spinal cord.

5.1.1 Stages of General Anaesthesia

The following are well defined stages produced by increasing the blood concentration of the anaesthesia. They are:

Stage I (Analgesia): This is the period from mild depression of higher neurons begins when from anaesthetic administration to the loss of consciousness. The patient progressively loses pain. This stage is also called stage of analgesia (cortical stage) and suitable for minor surgeries.

Stage II (Delirium): In this, the stage extends from the loss of consciousness to irregular and specific breathing. Respiration may be normal and regular after some time. There may be delirium, urination and uncontrolled muscular movement, laugh, vomit or struggle. Sometimes increased heart rate and blood pressure.

Stage III (Surgical Anaesthesia): In this stage excitement is lost and skeletal muscle relaxation is produced. Most types of surgeries are done in this stage.

Stage IV (Medullary Depression): Overdose of the anaesthetic drugs may cause this stage. Respiratory and circulatory failure occurs due to this.

5.1.2 Characteristics of General Anaesthetic Agents

An ideal general anaesthetic should possess the following characteristic features.

- It should be inert, potent and non-inflammable.
- It should be non-irritating to mucous membrane and able to produce rapid loss of consciousness along with prompt recovery.
- It should produce analgesia and muscle relaxation in addition to anaesthesia.
- It should not produce severe hypotension, nausea and vomiting.
- It should be compatible with adjuvant drugs used in anaesthesia and should not show any interactions or adverse effects.
- It should be stable to heat, light and alkaline, should be economical.

Mechanism of Action:

Generally act by depressing the neuronal activity in brain. Also exhibit different mechanism of action by acting on different location of brain during various stages explained by lipid and protein theory.

1. **Lipid Theory:** According to this, the more lipid soluble anaesthetics (general) concentrate near hydrophobic regions of neuronal cell membrane and causes swelling of these membranes. Due to this swelling, structure of membrane alters and thus it blocks the Na^+ channels. This inhibited the generation of action potential and produces anaesthesia. Meyer and Overton in 1901, correlated this theory of potency of general anaesthetics with their lipid solubility. Its general anaesthetic potency increases with the increase in partition coefficient of the compound.

2. **Protein Theory:** According to this theory, the anaesthetic moiety binds itself to the hydrophobic sites of protein molecules of neuronal cell membrane which cause alteration in the membrane function and produces anaesthesia.

5.1.3 Classification of General Anaesthetics

1. **Inhalation anaesthetics:** Halothane, Methoxyflurane, Enflurane, Sevoflurane, Isoflurane, Desflurane.

2. **Ultra short acting barbiturates:** Methohexital sodium, Thiamylal sodium, Thiopental sodium.

3. **Dissociative anaesthetics:** Ketamine hydrochloride.

5.2 INHALATION / VOLATILE ANAESTHETICS

They are generally administered by inhalation process and can be further divided into volatile liquids and gases.

5.2.1 Halothane

Chemically halothane is 2-bromo, 2-chloro, 1,1,1-trifluoroethane.

It produces a rapid onset of reaction without causing hypoxia. When given in combination with nitrous oxide the potency of drug increases and more potent than chloroform and ether. It is inflammable and thus safe to use and store.

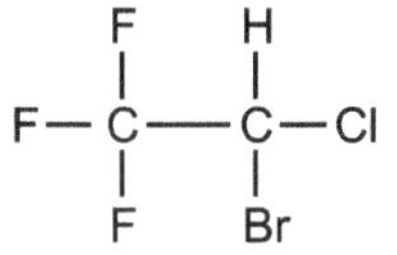

Halothane

Synthesis:

(a) From trichloro ethylene:

Trichloro ethylene

Halothane

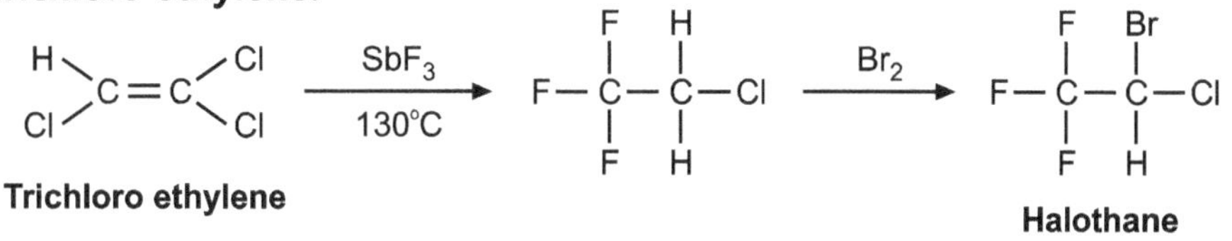

(b) From trichloro ethylene:

Trichloro ethylene

Halothane

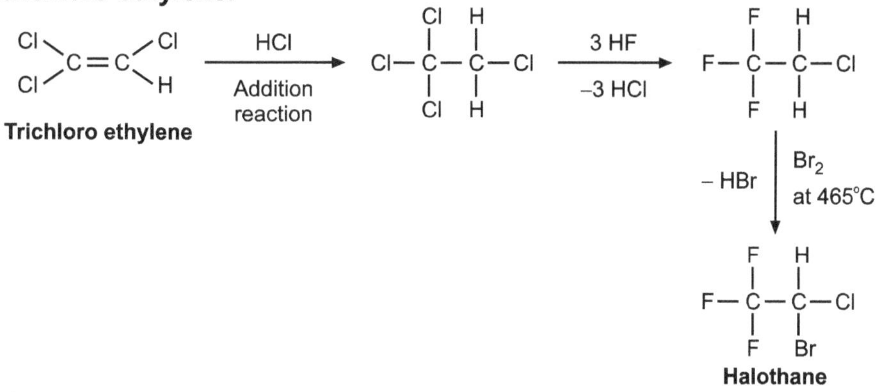

Side Effects:

1. It has a narrow margin of safety and a low incidence of hepatic necrosis.
2. It produces respiratory depression and hypotension.

5.2.2 Methoxyflurane

Chemically, methoxyflurane is 2,2-dichloro-1,1-difluoro-1-methoxyethane.

It is non-flammable, non-explosive and most potent of all inhalation anaesthetic. They are lipid soluble drugs. It is a colourless liquid with sweet odour.

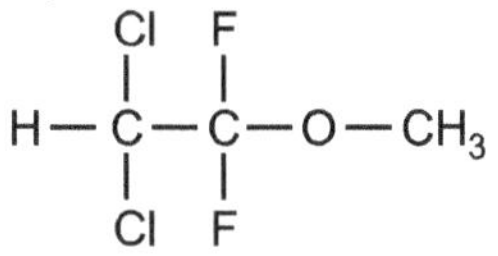

Methoxyflurane

Side Effects: It has a large blood gas partition coefficient and therefore has a slow induction and recovery phase. It may cause renal damage on prolonged use due to fluoride release.

5.2.3 Enflurane

Chemically, Enflurane is (2-chloro-1,1, 2-trifluroethyl) (difluromethyl) ether.

It is a clear, colourless, volatile liquid with pleasant hydrocarbon like odour. Soluble in water, miscible with organic solvent. Chemically it is extremely soluble.

$$H-\underset{\underset{F}{|}}{\overset{\overset{F}{|}}{C}}-O-\underset{\underset{F}{|}}{\overset{\overset{F}{|}}{C}}-\underset{\underset{H}{|}}{\overset{\overset{F}{|}}{C}}-Cl$$

Enflurane

Uses: Enflurane used in the treatment of Sotus Aathmoticas Ventricular Premature Complexes. Used for the induction and maintenance of general anaesthesia during surgery and cesarian section and during delivery.

Side Effects: (Acute) Nausea, vomiting, irritation of eyes, nose, throat, skin, Headache. (Chronic) Drowsiness, arrhythmias, respiratory depression, and liver/kidney dysfunction.

5.2.4 Sevoflurane

Chemically sevoflurane is 1,1,1,3,3,3-hexafluro-2(fluoromethoxy) propane.

It is a low boiling liquid with slight odour. Miscible with most organic solvents including fat and oils. Insoluble in water.

$$H-\underset{\underset{F_3C}{|}}{\overset{\overset{F_3C}{|}}{C}}-O-\underset{\underset{F}{|}}{\overset{\overset{F}{|}}{C}}-H$$

Sevoflurane

Uses: It is one of the most commonly used volatile anaesthetic agents. It is often used to put children on sleep for surgery by inhalation.

Side Effects: Nausea, vomiting, hypotension, agitation and cough.

5.2.5 Isoflurane

Chemically, isoflurane is (1-chloro-2,2,2-trifluroethyl) (difluoro methyl) ether. It is a clear, colourless, heavy liquid. Insoluble in water, soluble in ethanol and trichloroethylene. Also miscible in organic liquids including fats and oils.

1. It resembles isomer enflurane in properties.
2. It is non-flammable in air or oxygen.

$$F-\underset{\underset{F}{|}}{\overset{\overset{F}{|}}{C}}-\underset{\underset{H}{|}}{\overset{\overset{Cl}{|}}{C}}-O-\underset{\underset{F}{|}}{\overset{\overset{F}{|}}{C}}-F$$

Isoflurane

Uses: The depth of anaesthesia can be rapidly adjusted. Used for the induction and maintenance of general anaesthesia.

Side Effects: Respiratory depression, low B.P. and irregular heart beat.

5.2.6 Desflurane

Chemically, desflurane is 1,2,2,2-tetrafluoroethyl difluoromethyl ether.

It has a pungent odour, irritating and unpleasant to inhale and produce approvable incidence of salivation. Causes breath-holding, coughing or laryngospasm when given to conscious patient. It has a boiling point of 22.8°C.

Desflurane

Uses:

1. It is used to cause general anaesthesia by inhalation before or during the surgery in adults.

2. It has the most rapid onset and offset of all the volatile anaesthetic drugs used for general anaesthesia due to its low solubility in blood.

Side Effects: Bluish lips or skin, body ache, pain cough, running nose, blurred vision, dizziness, headache.

5.3 ULTRA SHORT ACTING BARBITURATES / NON-VOLATILE

They are non-volatile at room temperature and are administered by intravenous route. They are used to produce rapid unconsciousness for surgical and basal anaesthesia. These drugs induce anaesthesia during surgery which then maintained by inhalation anaesthetics. Sodium salts of methohexital and thiopental are the most commonly used barbiturates used to produce anaesthesia.

5.3.1 Methohexital Sodium

Chemically, it is methohexital sodium-1-methyl-5-allyl-5-(1-methyl-2-pentynyl). It is administered by intravenous route or intramuscular route and synthesis is as follows:

Methohexital

Synthesis:

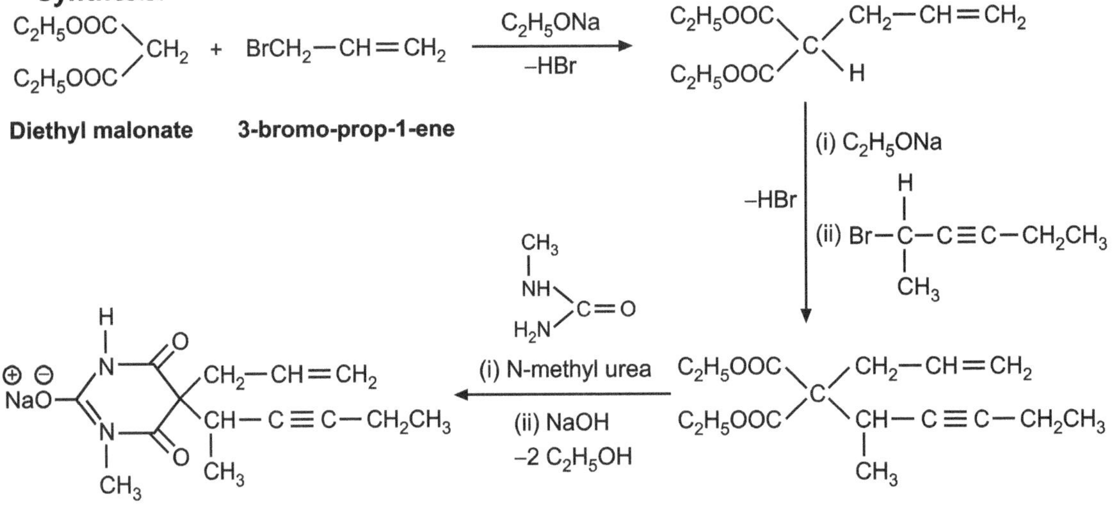

Diethyl malonate + 3-bromo-prop-1-ene $\xrightarrow[\text{–HBr}]{C_2H_5ONa}$ (allyl diethyl malonate)

(i) C_2H_5ONa
–HBr
(ii) $Br-\overset{CH_3}{\underset{\underset{CH_3}{|}}{\overset{|}{C}}}-C\equiv C-CH_2CH_3$

$\xleftarrow[\substack{\text{(ii) NaOH} \\ -2\,C_2H_5OH}]{\text{(i) N-methyl urea}}$

Methohexital sodium

Uses: It is used as a general anaesthetic and hypnotic drug for oral surgery, in gynaecological procedures, genito-urinary investigations and electro convulsive therapy. It is more potent than thiopentone sodium.

5.3.2 Thiamylal Sodium

Chemically thiamylal sodium is a salt of 5-allyl-5 (1-methyl butyl)-2- thiobarbiturate. It is highly hydrophobic thiobarbiturate having similar structural feature related to thiopental.

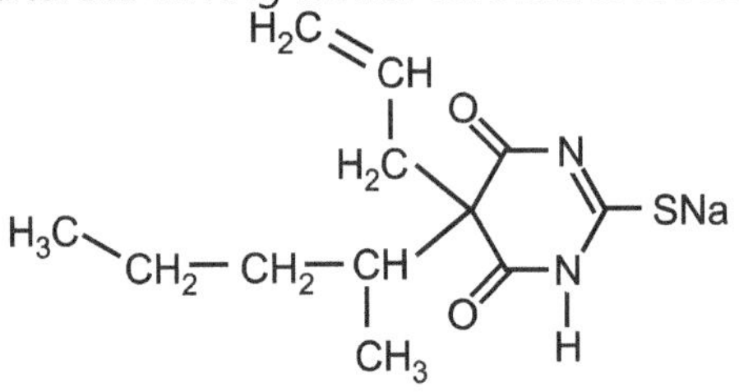

Thiamylal sodium

Uses: It is an intravenous anaesthetic drug used to induce drowsiness or sleep or psychological excitement (anxiety).

Side Effects: Coughing, sneezing, slow breathing, slow heart rate, shivering, cardiac arrhythmia.

5.3.3 Thiopental Sodium

Chemically thiopental sodium is a [5-Ethyl-4,6-dioxo-5-(pentan-2-yl)-1,4,5,6-tetrahydropyrimidin-2-yl]sulfanide sodium. It is used commonly in the induction phase of general anaesthesia, administered by IV route. It has a rapid onset of action and causes unconsciousness within 30-45 seconds.

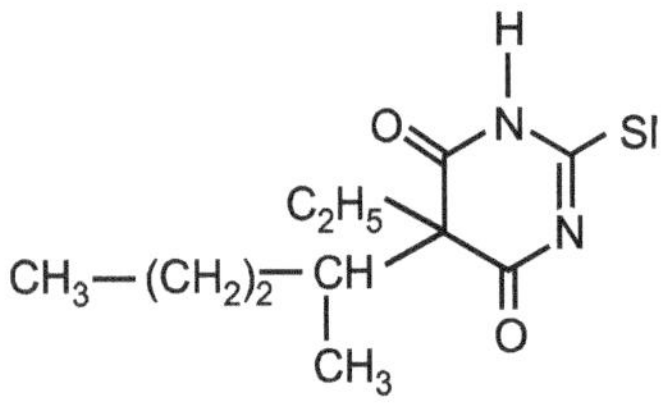

Thiopental sodium

Uses: Used in cesarean delivery. Also used in maintaining anaesthesia during surgery.

Side Effects: Reduce cardiac output, cause hypotension.

5.4 DISSOCIATIVE ANAESTHETIC

Dissociative anaesthesia is a state in which a patient feels dissociative completely from the surroundings. Dissociative anaesthesia is a class of hallucinogen, which distort perception of sight and sound and produce feelings of detachments – dissociation from the environment and self. This is done through reducing or blocking signals to the conscious mind from other parts of the brain. Many dissociative anaesthetic have general depressant effects and can produce sedation, respiratory depression analgesia and anaesthesia. Ketamine hydrochloride is the only drug used presently to produce this effect.

5.4.1 Ketamine Hydrochloride

Chemically, ketamine hydrochloride is (+) 2-(o-chlorophenyl)-2-methylaminocyclo-hexanone). It is a colourless crystalline solid compound with characteristic odour. Its melting point is 258°C.

Ketamine hydrochloride

Synthesis: Ketamine is prepared by Grignard reaction. In the presence of strong alkali, o-chlorobenzonitrile reacts with bromocyclopentane to give an epoxy compound which converts to an imine in the presence of methylamine. It then rearranges to give ketamine on heating with HCl.

o-chlorobenzonitrile   **Bromo-cyclopentane**   **2-(2-chlorophenyl-2-methoxy-1-oxaspiro[2,4]heptane**

Methyl amine
H_3C-NH_2

2-(2-chlorophenyl)-2-(methylamino)cyclohexanone Hydrochloride

Δ HCl
Rearrangement

2-((2-chlorophenyl)(methylimino)methyl)cyclopentanol Intermediate

Uses: It can be used as a general anaesthetic and an analgesic. It causes the relaxation of skeletal muscles.

Side Effects: Include agitation, confusion or hallucinations, low blood pressure and muscle tremors. Spasms of the larynx may occur sometimes.

5.5 NARCOTIC AND NON-NARCOTIC ANALGESICS

Narcotic analgesics were known as opioid narcotic analgesic drugs that relieve pain. These drugs bind to the opioid receptors located in the central and peripheral nervous system and cause numbness and a state of unconsciousness.

Classification of Analgesics:
1. **Natural compounds:** Morphine, codeine, papaverine.
2. **Semi-synthetic compounds:** Diacetylmorphine (Heroin), benzylmorphine, ethylmorphine.
3. **Synthetic compounds:** Fentanyl, pethidine, methadone, tramadol, propoxyphene hydrochloride (loperamide hydrochloride does not enter brain and thus lack of analgesic activity).

Mechanism of Action:

All opioid receptors are G-protein coupled receptors and inhibit adenylatecyclase. They are also involved in,
1. Postsynaptic hyperpolarization (increasing K^+ efflux).
2. Reducing presynaptic Ca^{++} influx thus inhibits neuronal activity.

Opioid receptors:

All opioid receptors are linked through G-proteins for the inhibition of adenylatecyclase. They facilitate the opening of potassium channels (causing hyperpolarisation) and inhibit opening of calcium channels (inhibiting transmitter release).

They are of four types of opioid receptors:
1. **μ-receptor:** μ-Receptors are thought to be responsible for most of the analgesic effects of opioids, and for some major unwanted effects. Most of the analgesic opioids are μ-receptor agonists. They are of two types:
   (a) **μ-1 receptor:** This is located outside the spinal cord. This receptor is responsible for the central interpretation of the pain.
   (b) **μ-2 receptor:** This is located throughout CNS and is responsible for respiratory depression, spinal analgesia, physical dependence and euphoria.
2. **σ-receptor:** σ-receptors are not true opioid receptors and its activity is not clear. It may regulate μ-receptor activity.
3. **δ-receptor:** δ-receptors are more important in the periphery and may also contribute to analgesia.
4. **κ-receptors:** κ-receptors contribute to analgesia at the spinal level and may elicit sedation and dysphoria, but produce relatively few unwanted effects and do not contribute to dependence.

5.6 MORPHINE AND RELATED DRUGS

Morphine is the major analgesic drug contained in crude opium. Morphine may be given by injection (intravenous or intramuscular) or as slow-release tablets. It is metabolized to morphine-6-glucuronide, which is most potent analgesic.

Analgesia, euphoria and sedation, respiratory depression and suppression of cough, nausea and vomiting, reduce gastrointestinal motility.

Side Effects: Addiction of drug is due to euphoric effect, overdose causes poisoning, coma and respiratory depression, dryness of mouth, mental clouding, vomiting, headache, fatigue, constipation etc.

The morphine molecule has the following important structural features:

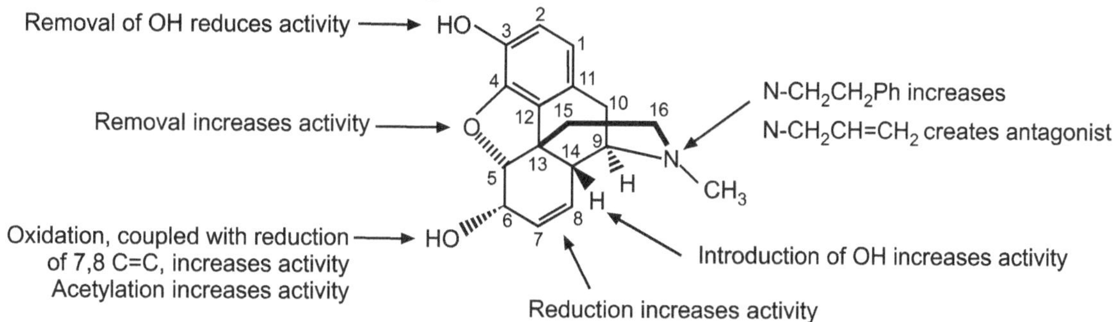

(+)-Morphine   **(−)-Morphine**

1. A rigid pentacyclic structure consisting of a benzene ring (A), two partially unsaturated cyclohexane rings (B and C), a piperidine ring (D) and a dihydrofuran ring (E). Rings A, B and C are the phenanthrene ring systems.

2. Ring A and its 3-hydroxyl group is an important structural feature for analgesic activity. Removal of the 3-OH group reduces analgesic activity by 10-fold.

3. Two hydroxyl functional groups, a C3-phenolic OH (pK$_a$ 9.9) and a C6-allylic OH.

4. An ether linkage between C4 and C5.

5. Unsaturation between C7 and C8.

6. A basic, 3°-amine function at position 17.

7. Five centres of chirality (C5, C6, C9, C13 and C14) with morphine exhibiting a high degree of stereoselectivity of analgesic action. Only (-)-morphine is active.

5.6.1 SAR of Morphine Analogues

1. Phenolic hydroxyl group at C3.

2. Alcoholic hydroxyl group at C6.

3. Alicyclic unsaturated linkage at C7–C8.

4.   Tertiary nitrogen.

5.   C14.

6.   Ether bridge.

Phenolic Hydroxyl Group at C3 (Ring A Analogues)

Ring A or Aromatic phenyl ring and its 3-hydroxyl group is an important structural feature for analgesic activity. Removal of the 3-OH group reduces analgesic activity by 10-fold.

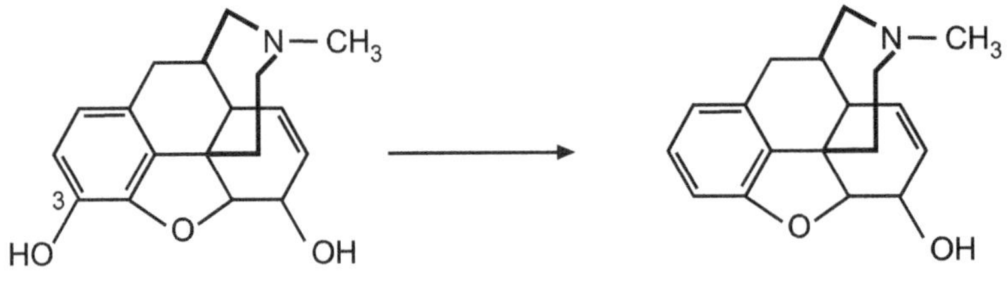

Morphine   **3-Deoxymorphine : RP = 0.1**

Altering the C-3 OH by etherification as shown by the derivatives below reduces narcotic analgesic activity.

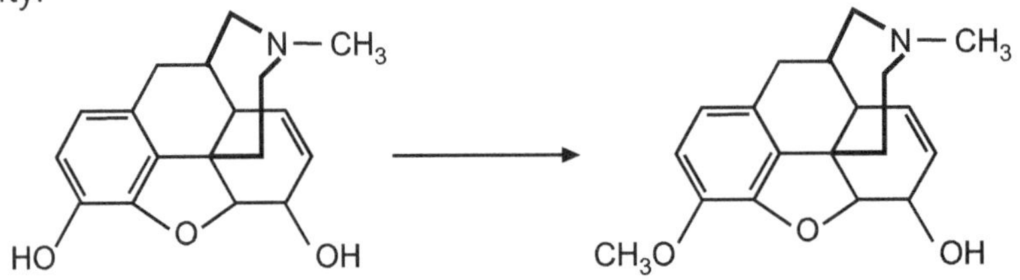

Morphine   **Codeine : RP = 0.15**

Esterification (acetylation) of both the 3- and 6-OH groups yields heroin, which is more lipophilic and more potent. The primary factor involved in increased analgesic potency is the increased lipophilicity and distribution to the CNS.

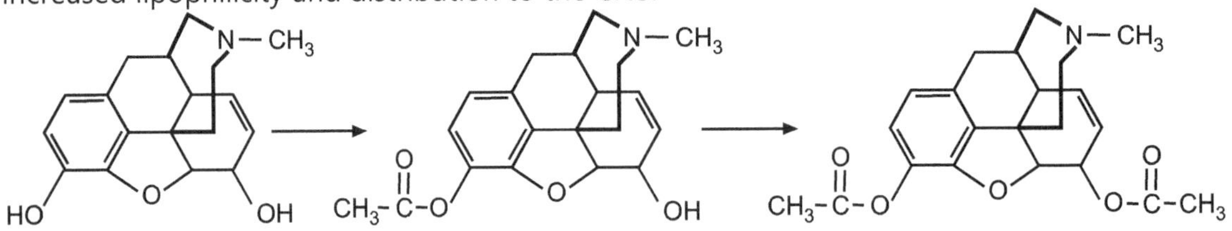

Morphine   **3-Acetylmorphine : RP > 1.0**   **Diacetylmorphine (Heroin) : RP = 2.0**

Heroin is much more potent than morphine but without respiratory depression effect. Acetyl groups are readily removed by metabolism to active morphine. It is not used because of additive nature. But in case of codeine conversion of the 3-OH to a 3-OCH$_3$, yields codeine, reduces activity to 15% of morphine.

Alcoholic Hydroxyl Group at C6 (Ring C Analogues)

The 6-OH of morphine is not required for analgesic activity as indicated by the relative potencies of the following morphine analogues.

Elimination of the 6-OH actually enhances activity. Etherification of this group with relatively small alkyl group also increases activity.

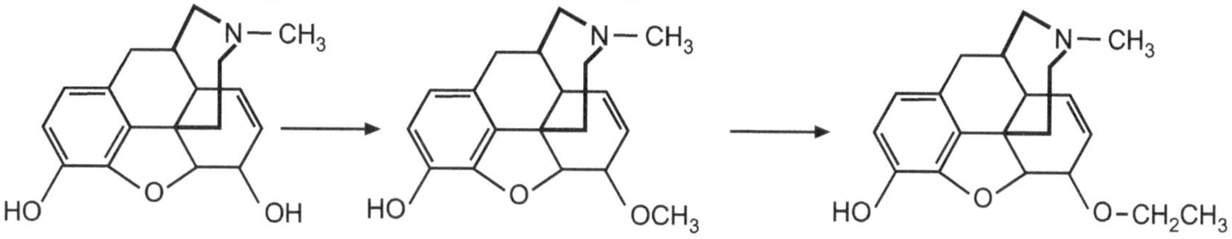

Morphine   **6-Methoxymorphine : RP = 5**   **6-Ethoxymorphine : RP = 2.5**

Oxidation of the 6-OH of dihydromorphine to yield hydromorphone further increases activity.

Oxidation of the 6-OH of morphine directly as in morphone (without reduction of the 7,8-double bond) does not significantly alter analgesic activity.

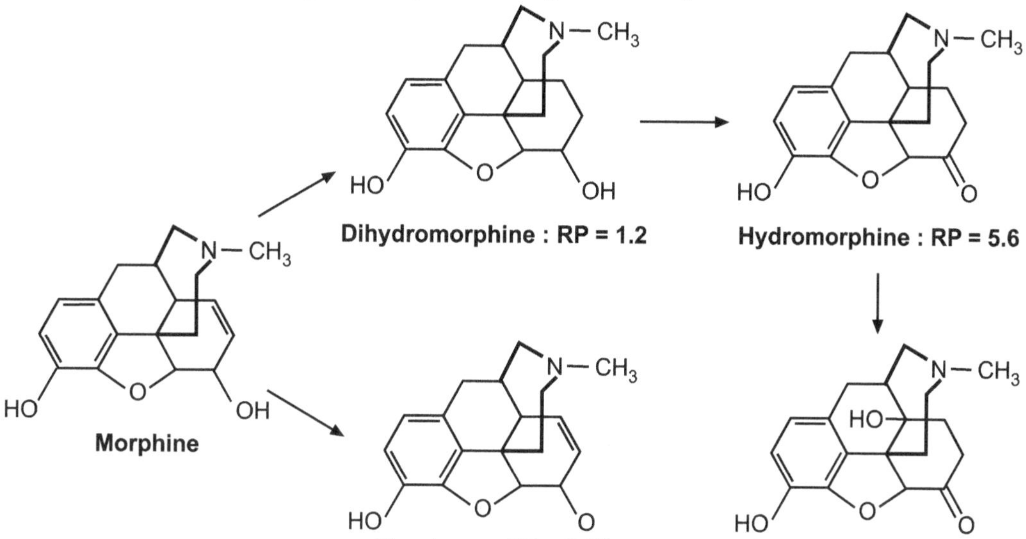

Dihydromorphine : RP = 1.2   **Hydromorphine : RP = 5.6**

Morphine

Morphone : RP = 0.66   **Oxymorphone : RP = 10**

In case of codeine, oxidation of 6-OH of dihydrocodeine as in hydrocodone results in a further increase in activity.

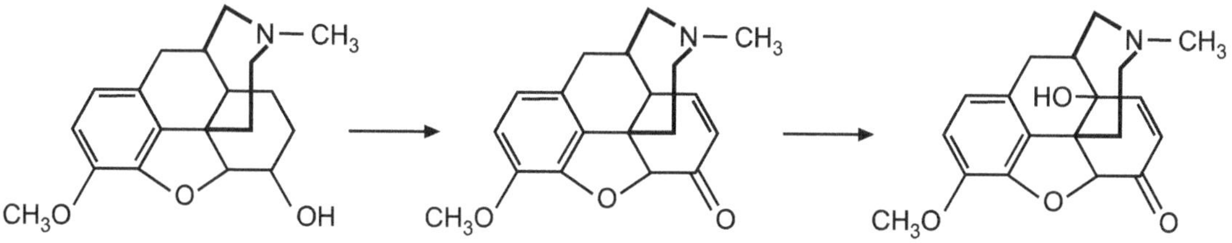

Dihydrocodeine : RP = 0.3   **Hydrocodone : RP = 0.7**   **Oxycodone : RP = 1.0**
(Codeine : RP = 1.15)   **(Codeine : RP = 5)**   **(Codeine : RP = 7)**

Hydrocodone is available in tablets and syrups and used as analgesic and anti-tussive activity. Oxycodone is available as tablets and capsules and used as analgesic and anti-tussive activity.

Alicyclic Unsaturated Linkage at C7–C8:

The 7,8-double bond of morphine also is not required for analgesic activity as indicated by the relative analgesic potency of dihydromorphine.

Substitution of a 14-OH group on the hydromorphone structure as in oxymorphone produces a further increase in analgesic activity (RP = 10).

Dihydromorphine : RP = 1.2

Dihydrocodeine : RP = 0.3
(Codeine : RP = 1.15)

Reduction of codeine's 7,8-double bond as in dihydrocodeine increases activity relative to codeine. 14-OH substitution produces a further increase in analgesic activity.

Oxymorphone : RP = 10

Tertiary Nitrogen (Ring D Analogues and the Tertiary Amine Function):

Replacement of morphine's N-methyl group by a hydrogen atom as in normorphine reduces analgesic activity to $1/8^{th}$ that of morphine, this decrease is due to increased polarity resulting in reduced blood brain barrier translocation to the CNS.

Replacement of morphine's N-methyl group with an allyl group ($-CH_2-CH=CH_2$), a methylcyclopropyl group or a methylcyclobutyl group results in opiate receptor antagonist activity.

Morphine

Normorphine

Morphine

Naloxone

C14 (Ring D Analogues):

The Thebaines: Adding a sixth ring across carbons 6 and 14 of the C ring of morphine yields thebaine compounds such as etorphine which are extremely potent analgesics. Replacement of the N-methyl group of the thebaine with a methylcyclopropyl group yields compounds with mixed agonist/antagonist or partial agonist activity.

Etorphine

Buprenorphine

Levorphanol

Epoxide Bridge:

Removal of 3,4 epoxide bridge in morphine structure is referred as morphinans, only laevo isomer possess opioid activity while the dextro isomer has useful antitussive activity.

5.6.2 Morphine Sulphate

Morphine is used primarily to treat both acute and chronic severe pain. It is also used for pain due to myocardial infarction and for labour pains. It acts directly on the central nervous system (CNS) to decrease the feeling of pain. It can be administered orally or by IV into a muscle, by injection under the skin, around the spinal cord, or rectally. Maximum effect is reached after about 20 minutes when given intravenously and after 60 minutes when given orally, last for 3-7 hours.

Morphine sulphate

Side Effects: Constipation, dizziness, perspiration, dry mouth, visual difficulty, itching, euphoria, restlessness, nervousness and excitement, addiction.

5.6.3 Codeine

Codeine is an opiate drug used to treat mild to moderate degrees of pain and also the pain associated with cough and diarrhoea. For more effects it has been combined with paracetamol or with non-steroidal anti-inflammatory drug.

Codeine $C_{18}H_{21}NO_3$

Side Effects: Vomiting, constipation, itchiness, light-headedness, and drowsiness, breathing difficulties and addiction. It is not recommended in children and pregnant women without consultation.

5.6.4 SAR of Phenyl (Ethyl) Piperidines / Meperidine Analogs

1. Replacement of C-4 phenyl group of meperidine by H, alkyl, aryl, aryl-alkyl and heterocyclic group decreases the analgesic activity.
2. Introduction of m-OH group on the phenyl ring increases the activity.
3. Presence of phenyl and ester group at 4th position of 1-methyl piperidine results in optimum activity.
4. Replacement of the carbethoxy group in Mepiridine by acyloxy group gave better analgesic as well as spasmolytic.
5. Replacement of phenyl group by phenylethyl derivative seems to be 3-times as active as Mepiridine.
6. The amino congener is 4 times more active (Anileridine). Enlargement of piperidine ring to 7-membered hexahydroazepine is less active but has low incidence of side effects. (e.g.) Proheptazine.
7. Contraction of piperidine ring to pyrrolidine gives more active compound but causes abuse liability (e.g) Alphaprodine and Procilidine.
8. In fentanyl, the phenyl and acyl groups are separated by nitrogen. It is 50 times stronger than morphine with minimal side effects.
9. Its short duration of action makes it well suited for use in anaesthesia. The C-3 methyl analog with an ester group at C-4 like lofentanil is 8400 times more potent than Meperidine as an analgesic. p-Chloroanalogloperamide cannot penetrate BBB sufficiently to produce analgesia. Diphenoxylate, a structural hybrid of Meperidine and Methadone is devoid of analgesic activity. It is effective in the treatment of diarrhoea.

5.6.5 Meperidine Hydrochloride

It is a narcotic analgesic used for the relief of most types of moderate to severe pain, including postoperative pain and the labour pain. R^3- ethyl carboxyl ester substitute increases the activity than morphine.

Meperidine hydrochloride

Side Effect: Prolonged use may lead to dependence of drug similar to morphine.

5.6.6 Anilerdine Hydrochloride

It is a synthetic analgesic drug and from piperidine class of analgesic agents. It differs from pethidine (meperidine) in that the N-methyl group of meperidine is replaced by an N-aminophenethyl group, which increases its analgesic activity.

Side Effects: Dizziness, perspiration, a feeling of warmth, dry mouth, visual difficulty, itching, euphoria, restlessness, nervousness and excitement.

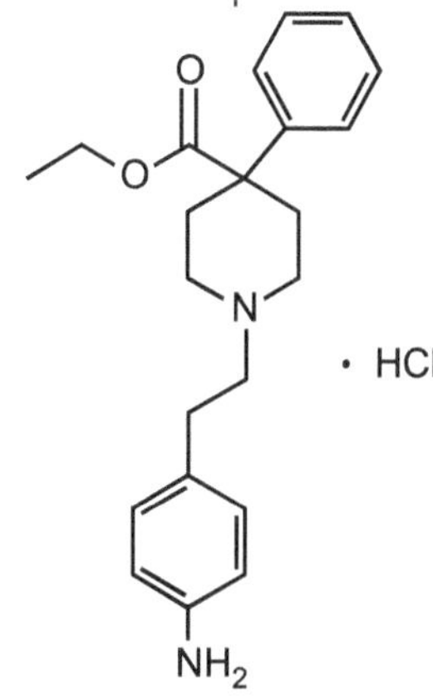

Anilerdine hydrochloride

5.6.7 Diphenoxylate Hydrochloride

Diphenoxylate are the derivatives of the phenylpepridines. It is used for the treatment of diarrhoea.

Diphenoxylate hydrochloride

Side Effects: It should not be given to children due breathlessness. It also includes numbness in the hands and feet, euphoria, depression, lethargy, confusion, drowsiness, dizziness, restlessness, headache, hallucinations, oedema, swollen gums, itchiness, vomiting, nausea, loss of appetite, and stomach pain.

5.6.8 Loperamide Hydrochloride

Loperamide can be taken orally. It is also used to treat diarrhoea in gastroenteritis, inflammatory and short bowel syndrome.

Loperamide hydrochloride

Side Effects: It causes abdominal pain, constipation, sleepiness, vomiting, and a dry mouth.

5.6.9 Fentanyl Citrate

Chemically, fentanyl citrate is N- (1-Phenylethyl-4-piperidinyl) propion-anilide citrate. It is structurally related to phenylpiperidines (e.g. *meperidine)*. R^1 is phenyl substituent group increases the activity 80 times than morphine.

Fentanyl citrate

Synthesis: N-(4-Piperidinyl) aniline is prepared by reductive amination of 4-piperidone and aniline, which is condensed with propionyl chloride to form amide. On N-alkylation with phenyl ethyl chloride, it gives fentanyl.

Use: Fentanyl citrate relieves moderate to severe breakthrough pain.

5.6.10 Methadone Hydrochloride

Chemically, Methadone hydrochloride is 6-(dimethylamino)-4,4-diphenyl-3-heptanone hydrochloride which is widely used as a narcotic analgesic, particularly in clinical treatment for the withdrawal of heroin addiction.

It is a synthetic drug and can be given orally. Its potency is similar to morphine but induces less euphoria and has a longer duration of action. The drug is bio transformed into inactive metabolites in the liver and is excreted in the urine.

Methadone hydrochloride

Synthesis: Methadone is prepared by reaction of 2,2-diphenyl-4-(dimethylamino)-pentane nitrile with an ethylmagnesium halide.

2,2-Diphenyl acetonitrile

2-Dimethylamino propyl chloride

Methadone

Side Effects: It can produce physical dependence like morphine, restlessness, nausea or vomiting, slow breathing, itchy skin, heavy sweating, constipation.

5.6.11 Propoxyphene Hydrochloride

Propoxyphene is a narcotic pain reliever. It is used to relieve mild to moderate pain.

Propoxyphene hydrochloride

Side Effects: Propoxyphene may be habit-forming. Not given to the patients having the history of addiction without consultation. It also causes confusion, hallucinations, nausea or vomiting, slow breathing.

5.6.12 Pentazocine

Pentazocine is used to treat moderate to severe pain. Chemically it is classed as a benzomorphan and it comes in two enantiomers.

(R)-Pentazocine　　　　　**(S)-Pentazocine**

Side Effects: High blood pressure, myocardial infarction, and respiratory depression.

5.6.13 Levorphenol Tartarate

Chemically, levorphenol is 3-hydroxy-*N*-methyl-morphinan. It is used to treat moderate to severe pain. It can be taken orally and has morphine-like analgesic activity.

Levorphenol tartarate

Side Effects: Hallucinations, drowsiness, dizziness, restlessness, headache, nausea.

5.7 NARCOTIC ANTAGONISTS

Replacement of morphine's N-methyl group with an allyl group ($-CH_2-CH=CH_2$), a methylcyclopropyl group or a methylcyclobutyl group results in the emergence of opiate receptor antagonist activity like naloxone HCl, naltrexone HCl and nalmefene respectively.

Morphine　　　　　**Antagonist activity**

$$R = -CH_2-CH=CH_2, \ -CH_2-C-C_3H_5, \ -CH_2-C-C_4H_7$$

5.7.1 Nalorphine Hydrochloride

Nalorphine is N-allylmorphine. In morphine tertiary nitrogen is attached to an allyl ($-CH_2CH=CH_2$) group. It is a white colored, odorless, crystalline powder. It darkens on exposure to light, so it has to to be kept in tight closed container. It is soluble in water, dilute alkali hydroxide solution but insoluble in chloroform and ether. It was used as an antidote to reverse opioid overdose and in a challenge test to determine opioid dependence.

Nalorphine is a mixed opioid agonist-antagonist with opioid antagonist and analgesic properties, used to treat narcotic-induced respiratory depression. It is administered by intravenous injection for treating the overdosage of morphine, pethidine, methadone and levorphanol.

Nalorphine

Side Effects: Dysphoria, anxiety, confusion, and hallucinations and therefore no longer used medically.

5.7.2 Levallorphan Tartarate

Levallorphan is available as tartarate salt, it is a white coloured, odourless, crystalline powder with melting point around 175°C. It is slightly soluble in water but insoluble in ether and chloroform. It acts as an antagonist of the μ-opioid receptor and as an agonist of the κ-opioid receptor. It blocks the effects of stronger agents like morphine with greater intrinsic activity. It is used the treatment of narcotic induced respiratory depression.

Levallorphan

Side Effects: Hallucinations, psychotomimetic effects, dysphoria, dizziness, disorientation, anxiety, confusion

5.7.3 Naloxone Hydrochloride

Naloxone is N-allyl-4, 5-epoxy-3, 14-dihydroxymorphinan-6-one. Naloxone is a derivative of 7, 8-dihydro-14-hydroxymorphinone having an allyl group at the nitrogen. Naloxone is administered by IV or IM and has a relatively short half-life (1 hour).

Replacement of the potent narcotic agonist oxymorphone's N-methyl group with an allyl group ($-CH_2-CH=CH_2$) gives naloxone. Naloxone is a pure antagonist without morphine like effects. It blocks the euphoric effect of heroin when is given before heroin.

Naloxone

Uses: Naloxone is a pure antagonist with no morphine like effects. It blocks the euphoric effect of heroin when given before heroin.

Side Effects: Nausea, vomiting, diarrhoea, stomach pain, fever, sweating, body aches, weakness, tremors or shivering, fast heart rate, pounding heart beats, increased blood pressure, restlessness.

5.8 ANTI-INFLAMMATORY AGENTS

Anti-inflammatory agents are the drugs used to reduce inflammation and the pain for the management of oedema and tissue damaging. They are also called as non-steroidal anti-inflammatory drugs (NSAIDs) and non-narcotic analgesics. It can be used topically, orally, parenteral for treating inflammation. Large number of drugs having anti-pyretic, anti-inflammatory, analgesic property and thus they can be used for the treatment of fever.

NSAIDs used in the treatment of rheumatoid arthritis, osteoarthritis (OA), acute gouty arthritis, ankylosing, spondylitis, dysmenorrhea and tissue damage resulting from inflammatory joint disease (arthritis). It has a wide range of therapeutic activity.

Characteristic Features of Anti-inflammatory Agents:

1. NSAIDs were also known as non-opioid analgesics, non-narcotic drugs as they do not interact with opioid receptors.
2. They do not have steroidal ring.
3. Their structure consists an acidic moiety (carboxylic or enols) attached to the planner aromatic functional group. Acidic group is essential for COX inhibitory activity and are the major binding group with plasma protein. Some contains polar linking group which is attached to planner moiety as an additional group.
4. Certain drugs have varying degree of activity against thrombocytes.
5. They act by exerting an inhibitory effect on cyclooxygenases (COX-I & COX-II), and thus inhibit the generation of various prostaglandins (PGs).
6. These drugs were metabolised and biotransferred by glucoronidation and then excreted via kidneys.

Classification of Anti-inflammatory Agents:

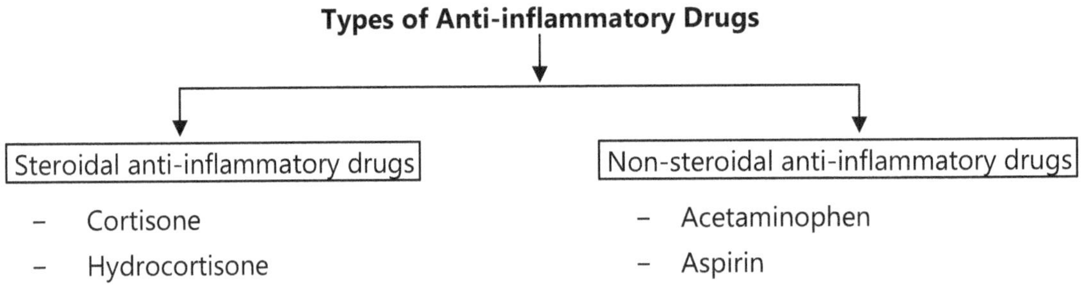

Mechanism of action of NSAIDs:

The major mechanism by which the NSAIDs shows their therapeutic effects (antipyretic, analgesic, and antiinflammatory activities) is inhibition of prostaglandin (PG) synthesis.

Specifically NSAIDs competitively inhibit cyclooxygenases (prostaglandin synthetase), the enzymes that catalyze the synthesis of cyclic endoperoxides from arachidonic acid to form prostaglandins. Generally, the NSAIDs inhibit both COX-1 and COX-2

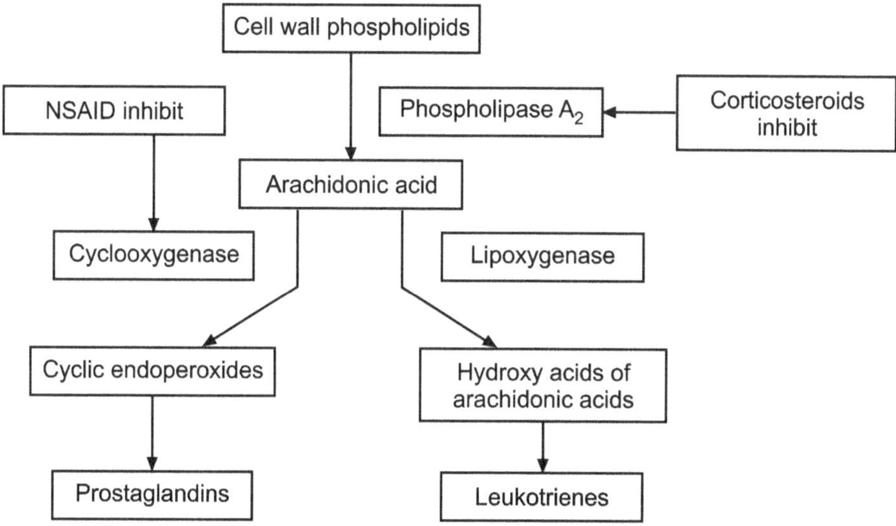

Biosynthetic pathways of prostaglandins and the mechanism of drugs which inhibit their production.

Further NSAIDs can be classified on the basis of their chemical structure as:

1. Salicylates: aspirin, sodium salicylate.
2. Propionic acids (Profens).
3. Aryl and heteroarylacetic acids.
4. Anthranilates (Fenamates).
5. Oxicams ("Enol Acids").
6. Phenylpyrazolones.
7. Anilides.

5.8.1 Salicylates

They are the derivatives of 2-hydroxybenzoic acid and used as a sodium salt. It has analgesic, anti-pyretic and anti-inflammatory activity.

Mechanism of Action: They act by inhibiting the biosynthesis of prostaglandins at the cyclooxygenase stage, thus blocking the formation of potent platelet aggregating factor, thromboxane A$_2$ (TX A$_2$). These drugs are mainly COX-1 selective and bound with higher affinity to COX-1. Some of the therapeutic actions of aspirin and related drugs as they inhibit COX-1 used to treat headache, discomfort, fever, muscle pain and aches and common cold.

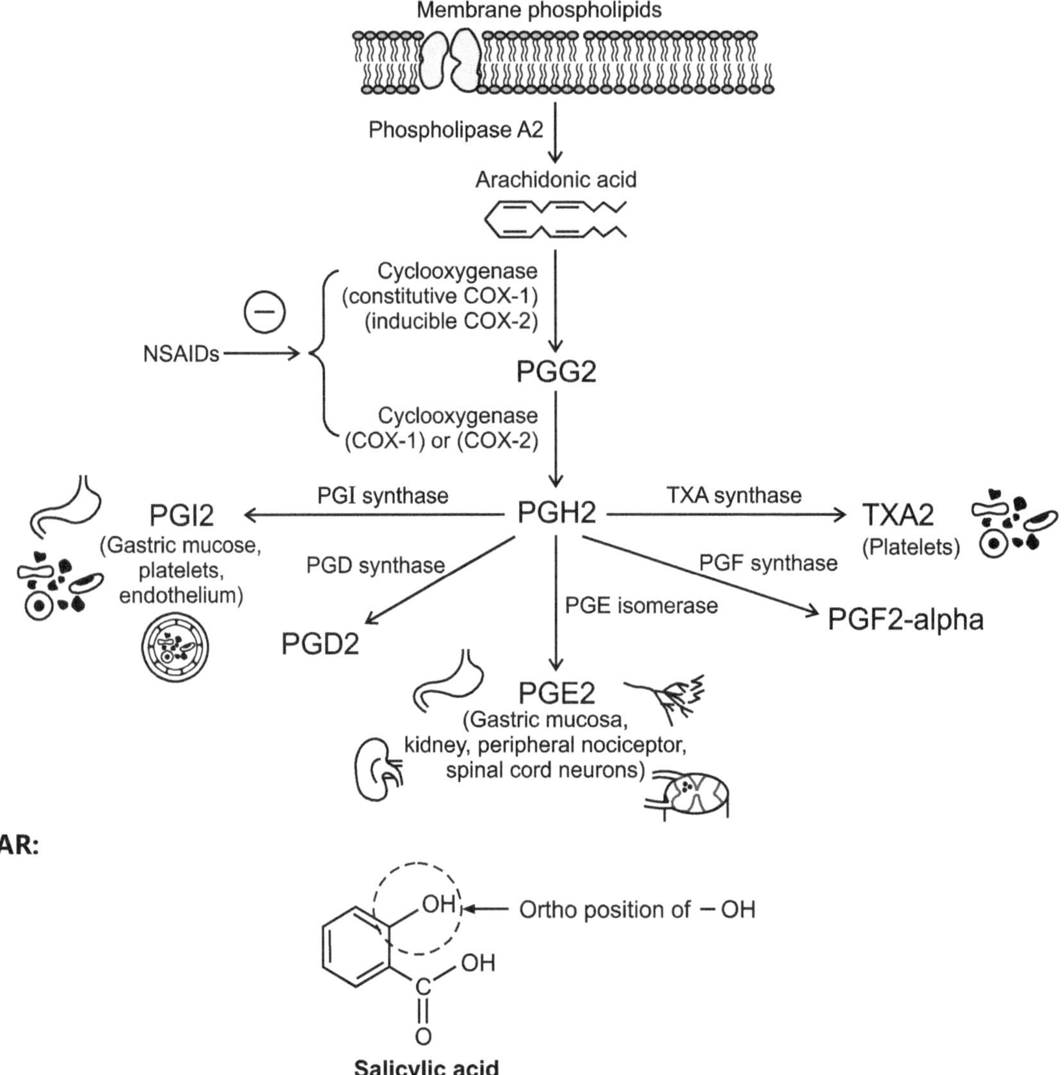

SAR:

Salicylic acid

- COOH functional group at position −C1 and −OR group at −C2 is essential for the anti-inflammatory activity of salicylic acid derivatives (salicylates).
- Replacement/substitution of COOH group may decrease or abolish the anti-inflammatory activity. It may show some analgesic activity. e.g, Salicylamide.
- Substitution of −OR group by −OH group at −C2 position increases the activity but decreases if placed at −C3, −C5 (meta) and −C4 (para) position.

Disulfinal

- Aryl group at −C5 position increases activity. Substitution by halogen or alkyl groups on aryl ring also increases the activity. e.g. Disulfinal.

5.8.2 Sodium Salicylate

Chemically, it is 2-hydroxy benzoate.

Sodium salicylate

Sodium salicylate is sodium 2-hydroxybenzenecarboxylate. It occurs as a white, crystalline powder or small, colourless crystals or shiny flakes. It is freely soluble in water, sparingly soluble in alcohol and practically insoluble in ether. It should be stored in an airtight container and protected from light.

Uses: Sodium salicylate is employed for the relief of pain, rheumatic fever and symptomatic treatment of gout.

5.8.3 Aspirin (Acetylsalicylic Acid)

It is an acetyl derivative of salicylic acid and was introduced by Dreser in 1899. Aspirin occurs as colourless crystals or powder. It is slightly soluble in water and soluble in alcohol, chloroform, ether and glycerine. Aspirin is stable in dry air but in the presence of moisture, it hydrolyses slowly into salicylic acid and acetic acid. Aspirin is acidic and produces effervescence with carbonates and bicarbonates.

Acetylsalicylic acid

Use: Aspirin is used as an antipyretic, analgesic and anti-rheumatic.

Synthesis: It is an esterification reaction in which the reaction between the hydroxyl groups of salicylic acid reacts with acetic anhydride to form an ester in the presence of an acid as a catalyst.

Salicylic acid   **Acetic anhydride**   **Acetylsalicylic acid**

5.8.4 Propionic Acids Derivatives (Profens)

Some NSAIDs were derived from arylacetic acids, known as the "profens" e.g., ibuprofen. These agents are all strong organic acids and form water soluble salts with alkaline reagents. The arylpropionic acids are characterized by the general structure Ar-CH(CH$_3$)-COOH which confirms to the required general structure.

Mechanism of Action: They are COX-1 inhibitors. Some compounds like naproxen appears to be more COX-2 inhibitors as compared to others.

Uses: For rheumatoid arthritis, osteoarthritis, analgesic and antipyretic. They should not be used during pregnancy or nursing. They produce less GI ulceration than the salicylates.

SAR:

- α-CH$_3$ substituent present in the structure increases cyclooxygenase inhibitory activity and reduces toxicity of the profens.
- The α-carbon in these compounds is chiral and the S-(+)-enantiomer of profens is more potent cyclooxygenase inhibitor.

General structure:

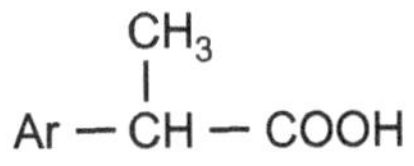

$$\overset{\displaystyle CH_3}{\underset{\displaystyle |}{Ar - CH - COOH}}$$

General structure of profen

5.8.5 Ibuprofen

Ibuprofen: It is a non-steroidal anti-inflammatory drug (NSAID), used for treating pain, fever, and inflammation.

Mechanism of Action: Ibuprofen is a non-selective, reversible inhibition of the cyclooxygenase enzymes COX-1 and COX-2 (coded for by PTGS1 and PTGS2, respectively).

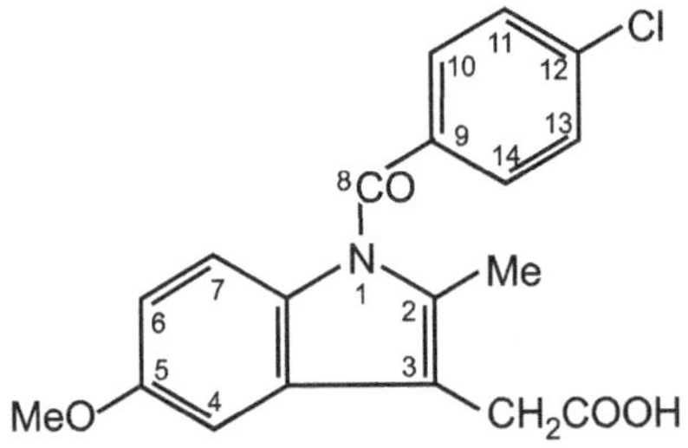

SAR

- The carboxyl group is essential for antiinflammatory activity.
- Presence of methoxy (position 5) group on the ring (5 or 6), methyl (2), dimethyl amino group (5) in indole moiety of indomethacin exhibit activity.
- Presence of chlorine or fluorine or CF3 groups at para position of phenyl group also exhibit anti-inflammatory activity.

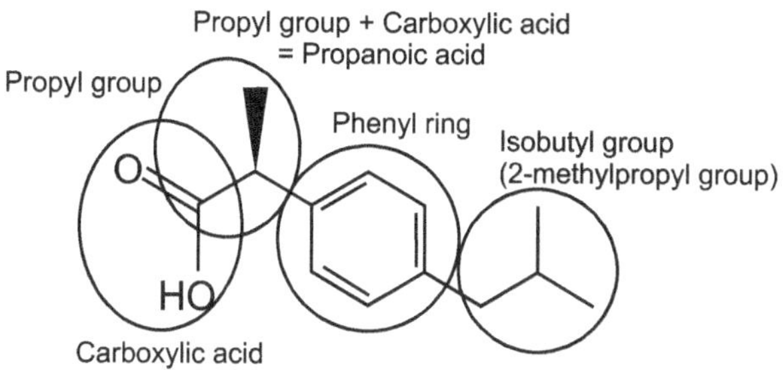

Synthesis of Ibuprofen: Two methods to obtain ibuprofen

1. **The Boot process:** The Boot process is an older commercial process developed by the Boot Pure Drug Company.

2. **The Hoechst process:** The Hoechst process is a newer process developed by the Hoechst Company. While the Hoechst process, with the assistance of catalysts.

Ibuprofen synthesis begins with isobutylbenzene and use Friedel-Craft's acylation.

Uses: In the treatment of rheumatoid arthritis, osteoarthritis, analgesic and antipyretic. It should not be used during pregnancy or nursing as it can enter fetal circulation and breast milk. It has less GI ulceration than the salicylates.

5.8.6 Naproxen

Chemically, Naproxen is naphthyl 6-methoxyisopropionic acid. It is a non-steroidal anti-inflammatory, antirheumatic, analgesic, antidysmenorrhoeal and vascular headache suppressant.

Naproxen

Naproxen is having (partly) an ability to inhibit COX-1 and COX-2. It irreversibly blocks the enzyme cyclooxygenase (prostaglandin synthase), which catalyzes the conversion of arachidonic acid to endoperoxide compounds and decreases the formation of prostaglandins.

Aryl and Heteroarylacetic Acid Derivatives: These compounds are the derivatives of acetic acid, but substituent at -C2 position is a heterocycle or carbo cycle. This does not alter the acidic properties of compounds of this group.

These NSAIDs can be further sub-classified as:

(a) Indene and indoles

(b) Pyrroles

(c) Oxazoles

General Structure:

General structure of aryl acetic acid

SAR:

- COOH group is essential for the activity. Replacement of this group diminishes or abolishes the activity.
- Increase in acidity of COOH group will increase the anti-inflammatory activity. Decrease in COOH acidity decreases the activity.
- Presence of indole ring is necessary for the activity. Substitution at C5 position (R2) by fluro, methyl, dimethylamino, alkoxy or acetyl group increases the activity. Alkyl group at C2 position increases activity as compared to aryl groups. Substitution at acetic acid chain gives compounds of greater activity. e.g, Indomethacin, sulindac, ketorolac,
- Presence of methoxy at -C5 position group on the ring, methyl at C2 position, dimethyl amino group at C5- position in indole moiety of indomethacin exhibit activity.
- Presence of chlorine or fluorine or CF_3 groups at para position of phenyl group also give anti-inflammatory activity.

Indomethacin

Etodolac

Sulindac

5.8.7 Indomethacin

Chemically, indomethacin is 1-(p-chlorobenzoyl)-5-methoxy-2-methylindole-3-acetic acid. It consists of benzene ring fused to indole ring. Indomethacin is available as white to yellow crystalline powder. It is practically soluble in water.

Structure-activity Relationship (SAR):

- The carboxyl group is essential for anti-inflammatory activity.
- Presence of methoxy (position 5) group on the ring (5 or 6), methyl (2), dimethyl amino group (5) in indole moiety of indomethacin exhibit activity.
- Presence of chlorine or fluorine or CF_3 groups at para position of phenyl group also exhibit anti-inflammatory activity.

Sulindac

Indomethacin

Side Effects: The most frequent side effects are peptic ulcer, blood disorders and gastrointestinal.

5.8.8 Sulidac

(Arylalkanoic acid Derivative): Chemically, it is 5-fluro-2 methyl [(4 methyl sulphinyl) phenyl methylene] indene-3-acetic acid. It is a yellowish crystalline powder. Very slightly soluble in water, soluble in methylene chloride and dilute solution of alkali hydroxides, sparingly soluble in alcohol.

Uses: It has an analgesic, anti-inflammatory activity; it is usually employed in the treatment of rheumatic and muscular skeletal disorder, acute gout arthritis and osteoarthritis.

Side Effects: Affect CNS and gastrointestinal irritations.

5.8.9 Tolmetin

It is a non-steroidal anti-inflammatory drug (NSAID) of heterocyclic acetic acid derivative class. It acts by reducing the levels of prostaglandins and thus reduced inflammation.

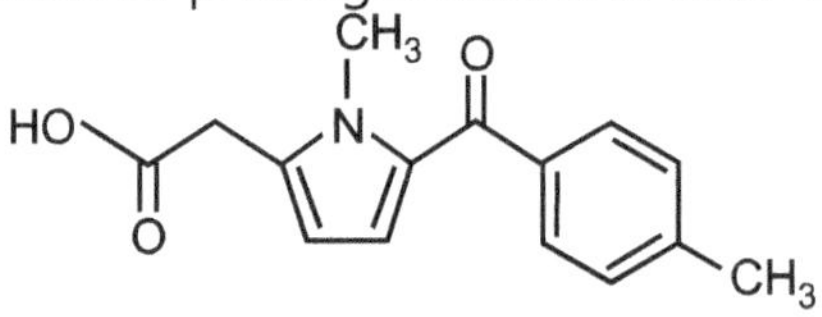

Tolmetin

Uses: To reduce hormones that cause pain, swelling, tenderness, and stiffness in conditions such as osteoarthritis and rheumatoid arthritis, including juvenile rheumatoid arthritis.

Side Effects: GI irritations, ulcer.

5.8.10 Pyrrolesarylacetic Acids

Ketorolac: It does not have benzylic methyl group, thus its half-life is about (4-6 hours) as it is not susceptible to oxidation. It is formulated for oral and IM administration showing good oral activity with primarily analgesic activity along with anti-inflammatory activity and antipyretic actions.

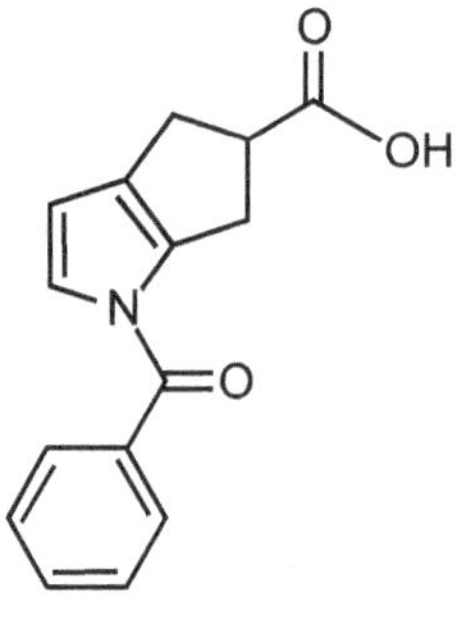

Ketorolac

Uses: In the management of post-operative pain.

Side Effects: Stomach pain, GI irritations, ulcer.

Oxazoles Arylacetic Acids: In 1993, oxaprozin was introduced having a non-selective COX inhibition activity. It differs from indomethacin and other compounds in the substitution of the propionic acid at the C3-position rather than at the C2-position.

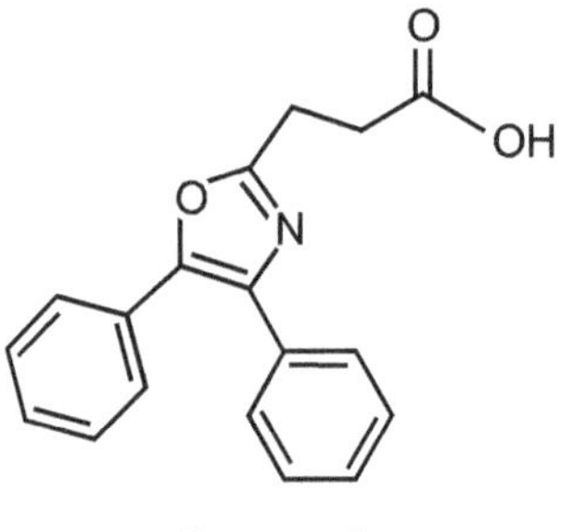

Oxaprozin

Uses: In the treatment of pain associated with surgery.

Side Effects: Vomiting, nausea, GI irritations, ulcer.

Anthranilates (Fenamates): (Anthranilic Acid Derivatives)

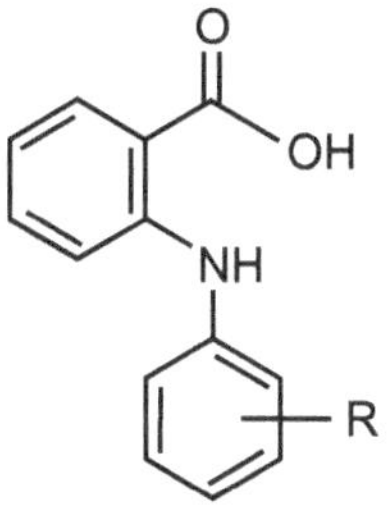

General anthranilate structure 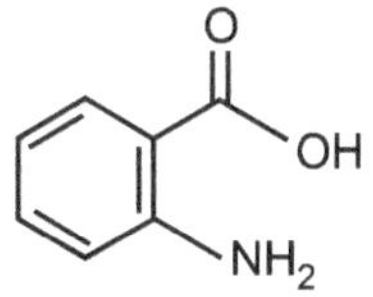   **Anthranilic acid**

SAR:

- They are N-aryl substituted derivatives of anthranilic acid.
- These compounds have small alkyl or halogen substituent at the C2', C3' and/or C6' position of the N-aryl moiety are 25 times more potent than mefenamate.
- Presence of –NH moiety is essential for the activity. Substitution by ether, thioether, ketonic, methylene or sulphur group decreases the activity.

Mechanism of Action: They are non-COX selective and have anti-inflammatory with some analgesic and antipyretic activity. The anthranilates are used as mild analgesic and occasionally to treat inflammatory disorders. Diclofenac is used for rheumatoid arthritis, osteoarthritis and post-operative pain and the utility of this class of agents is limited by a number of adverse reactions including nausea, vomiting, diarrhoea, ulceration, headache, drowsiness and hematopoietic toxicity.

Mefanamic Acid: Chemically, it is N-2,3-xylylanthranilic acid. It produces analgesic activity centrally and peripherally.

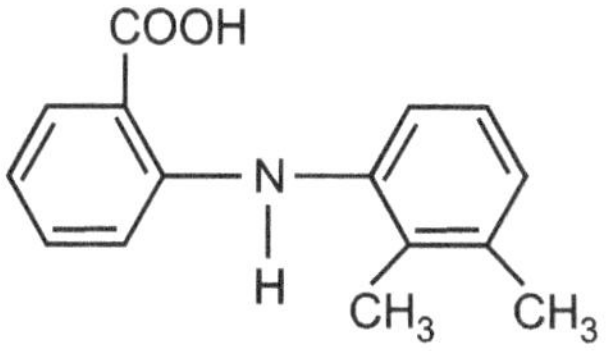

Mefenamic acid

Synthesis: Mefenamic acid can be prepared by condensing 2,3-xylidine with 2-chlorobenzoic acid aunder acidic conditions.

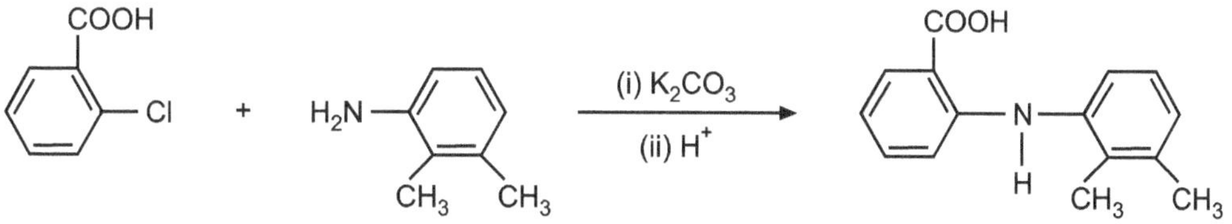

2-Chlorobenzoic acid   **2, 3-Xylidine**   **Mefenamic acid**

Uses: Mefenamic acid is used as an analgesic for the short-term relief from dysmenorrhoea.

Side Effects: Nausea vomiting, diarrhoea, ulceration, headache, drowsiness and hematopoietic toxicity.

Meclofenamate sodium: it is an anthranilic acid derivative. Chemically it is sodium (2,6-dichloro-3-methyl phenyl amino) benzoate. It is an anti-inflammatory drug for oral administration. Freely soluble in water. Meclofenamate capsule contains 50 mg or 100 mg.

Meclofenamate sodium

Uses: Meclofenamate is given for the relief of mild to moderate pain in acute and chronic rheumatoid, arthritis, osteo-artheritis. In the primary treatment of dysmenorrhoea and for the treatment of idiopathic heavy menstrual blood loss.

Contraindication: Meclofenamate sodium should not be used in those patients who have previously exhibited hypersensitivity to these drugs. Greater potential for cross sensitivity to aspirin or other non-steroidal anti-inflammatory drugs. It should not be given to those patients who show drug induce symptoms of bronchospasm, allergic rhenotix or urticarial.

Side Effects: Abdominal pain, oedema, urticaria, pruritis, headache, nausea, dizziness, tinnitus, blurred vision.

Diclofenac Sodium: Chemically, it is sodium [0-(2,6-dichloroanilino) phenyl] acetate. It acts (COX-2) as inhibitors with more potency than COX-1 inhibitors and have a lower GI irritations than aspirin.

Uses: As an anti-inflammatory, antipyretic, and analgesic agent.
Side Effects: Nausea, vomiting, ulceration, headache.
Oxicams (Enol Acid): They are the 4-hydroxybenzothiazine. The acidity of compound is because of the 4-OH which was stabilized by intramolecular hydrogen bonding to the amide N-H group, they were ionized at physiologic pH, it is required for COX inhibitory activity.

Piroxicam

Uses: In the treatment of rheumatoid, arthritis and osteoarthritis.
Side Effects: Nausea, vomiting, ulceration, headache.

Phenylpyrazolones: Chemically, it is 1-aryl-3,5 pyrazolidinedione structure. The presence of a proton which is situated α to two electron withdrawing carbonyl groups renders these compounds acidic. The pK_a for phenylbutazone is 4.5. Oxyphenbutazone is hydroxylated metabolite of phenylbutazone.

Phenylbutazone: They are the anti-inflammatory drugs, also possess some analgesic and antipyretic activities. They also have mild uricosuric activity.

Phenylbutazone

Uses: Phenylbutazone is used in the treatment of rheumatoid arthritis and osteoarthritis.

Side Effects: Include GI irritation, Na^+ and H_2O retention and blood dyscariasis. Therapy should be limited to 7-10 days due to development of bone marrow depression.

Antipyrine: Chemically it is 2, 3-dimethyl-1-phenyl-3-pyrazolin-5-one. It was one of the first synthetic compounds to be used in medicine. It is a colourless, crystalline white powder. It is odourless and having slightly bitter taste. It is freely soluble in water, alcohol, and chloroform.

Antipyrine

Uses: Analgesic, anti-inflammatory and antipyretic activities.

Side Effects: Include GI irritation, swelling, vomiting.

Anilides: The anilides are simple acetamides of aniline. It may or may not have a 4-hydroxy or 4-alkoxy group. It do not possess the carboxylic acid functionality and therefore they are the neutral drugs and possess little inhibitory activity against cyclooxygenase.

SAR:

- Esterification of phenolic group using methyl or propyl groups produces more side effects as compared to ethyl derivatives.
- Presence of substituents reduces basicity of nitrogen and thus decreases pharmacological activity of the drug.

General structure for anilides

Mechanism of Action: They are different from other NSAIDs in their mechanism of action. They act as scavengers of hydro-peroxide radicals (hydro-peroxide radicals are generated after injury). These radicals have a stimulating effect on cyclooxygenase. The concentration of hydro-peroxides at sight of injury and inflammation is high. Thus they do not have anti-inflammatory action. They are only capable of suppressing cyclooxygenase activity in areas which are not inflamed. The lack of an acidic group and COX inhibitory activity made anilides to have less gastric irritation, ulceration, and respiratory effects and little effect on platelets (no increase in clotting).

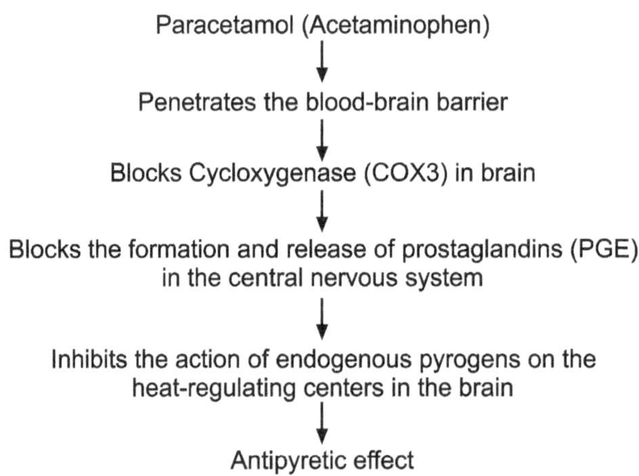

Acetaminophen (paracetamol)   **Phenacetin**

Acetaminophen: (Paracetamol): Chemically, it is N-acetyl-p-aminophen. It is a metabolite of phenacetin. It inhibits the cyclooxygenase enzyme centrally but has a less effect peripherally.

Mechanism of action of Paracetamol

Paracetamol (Acetaminophen)

↓

Penetrates the blood-brain barrier

↓

Blocks Cycloxygenase (COX3) in brain

↓

Blocks the formation and release of prostaglandins (PGE)
in the central nervous system

↓

Inhibits the action of endogenous pyrogens on the
heat-regulating centers in the brain

↓

Antipyretic effect

Uses: Analgesic and anti-pyretic activity.

Side Effects: Liver toxicity in chronic alcoholics.

> **Phenacetin:** Chemically, it is p-ethoxyacetanilide. It was introduced in 1885 to medicine. It causes haemolytic anaemia and meth-haemoglobinanemia. Its use has declined because of its adverse effects, which include increased risk of certain cancers and kidney damage. It is metabolized as paracetamol (acetaminophen).

Uses: Analgesic and anti-pyretic activity.

Side Effects: Include GI irritation.

QUESTIONS

1. Classify general anaesthetics with examples. Outline the synthesis of methoxy flurane and halothane.

2. What are general anaesthetics? Give its classification and outline the synthesis of methohexital sodium

3. Explain the importance of anaesthetics.

4. Write a note on inhalation anaesthetics.

5. Write briefly on ultra short acting barbiturates. Write a note on dissociative anaesthetics.

6. Outline the synthesis of naphazoline

7. Write the structure and uses of thiopental sodium and methohexital sodium.

8. Outline the synthesis of glutethimide sodium.

9. Write the structure and uses of ketamine hydrochloride.

10. What are analgesic? Classify analgesic with example. Outline the synthesis of Mefenamic acid and Ibuprofen.

11. Discuss the structural and nuclear modifications of morphine

12. What are non-narcotic analgesics? Give their detailed classification. Give the synthesis of any two agents.

13. What are anti-inflammatory agents? Classify them. Discuss the mechanism of action and give the synthesis of any two agents.

14. What are non-steroidal anti inflammatory drugs? Classify those giving structures. Give the synthesis of Ibuprofen and Oxyphenbutazone.

15. Outline the synthesis of Diphenhydramine and Pheniramine.

16. Write a note on narcotic antagonists with suitable examples.

17. Explain the chemistry and peripheral modifications of narcotic agents.

18. Give the classification of anti-inflammatory agents with example and outline the synthesis of phenacetin.

19. Write briefly on aniline and p-Aminophenol derivatives.

20. Give an account of chemistry of narcotic antagonist.

21. Outline the synthesis and uses of Oxyphenbutazone and Mefenamic acid.

22. Outline the synthesis and uses of Acetaminophen and Ibuprofen.

23. Write a note on morphine antagonist.

24. Write a note on salicyclic acid derivatives.

25. What are antitussive agents? Give the structure and uses of any two such agents.

✱✱✱